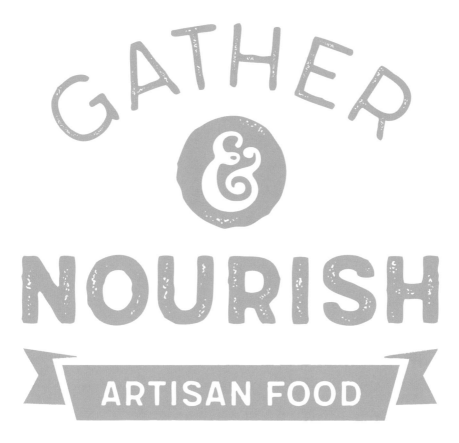

GATHER & NOURISH

ARTISAN FOOD

THE SEARCH FOR WELL-BEING AND
SUSTAINABILITY IN THE MODERN WORLD

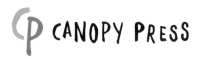

CANOPY PRESS

First published in the United Kingdom, 2019, by Canopy Press.
An imprint of 3dtotal Publishing.

Address: 3dtotal.com Ltd, 29 Foregate Street, Worcester, WR1 1DS, United Kingdom.
Correspondence: publishing@3dtotal.com
Website: canopy-press.com

ISBN: 978-1-909414-85-3

Printing and binding: Gomer Press, UK | gomer.co.uk

Visit canopy-press.com for a complete list of available book titles.

Managing Director: Tom Greenway
Studio Manager: Simon Morse
Assistant Manager: Melanie Robinson
Lead Designer: Imogen Williams
Publishing Manager: Jenny Fox-Proverbs
Template and cover design: Matthew Lewis
Layout: Joseph Cartwright
Illustrations: Marisa Lewis

Back cover photographs (from top to bottom):
© Willy's Ltd; © Beau Cacao; © Big Island Coffee Roasters;
© David De Vleeschauwer, www.classetouriste.com

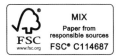

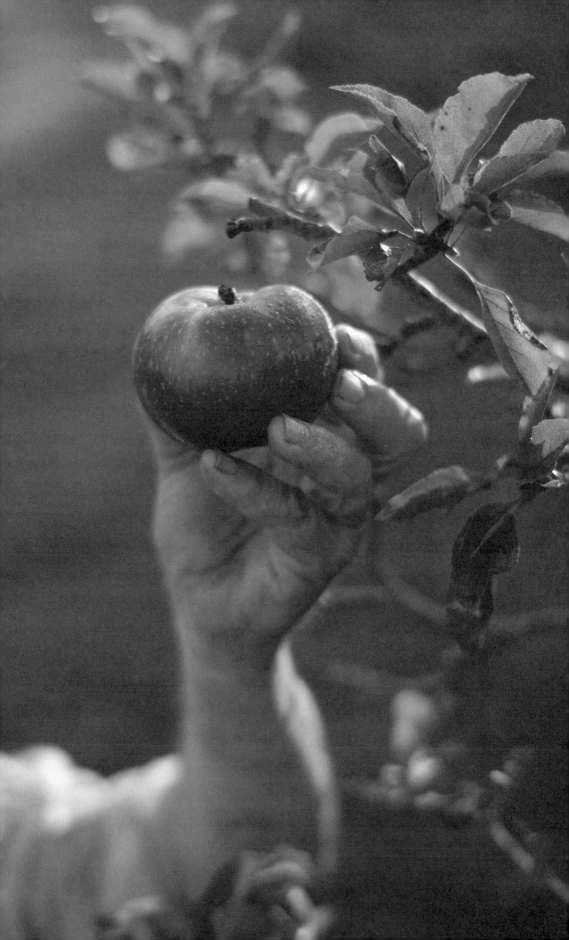

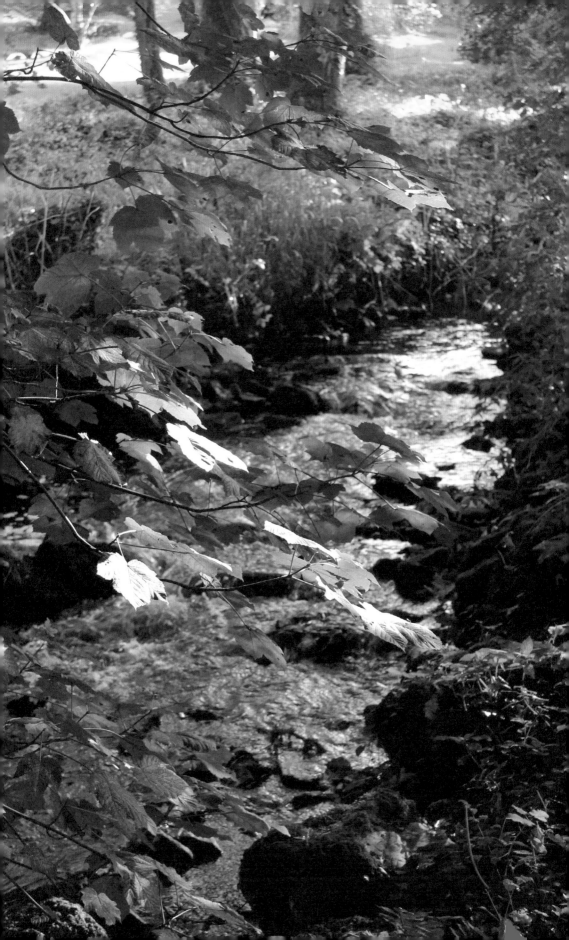

"Relating to your own gut, or to the planet around you, is the same action, and requires the same rules of engagement: Love it. Feed it. Don't poison it"

Shann Jones, Co-Director
of Chuckling Goat

CANOPY PRESS

An imprint of 3dtotal Publishing, Canopy Press was established in 2018 to create books focused on traditional crafts, lifestyle, and the environment. With an interest in enjoying the simple things in life, Canopy Press aims to build awareness around sustainable living, a mindful approach to arts and crafts, and an appreciation of the earth we dwell on.

Marrying great aesthetics with enlightening stories from real people, our *Search for Well-being and Sustainability in the Modern World* series presents an insight into heritage crafts and artisan food, and their revival and survival in the modern world. Visit our website and follow us on Instagram to stay up to date with forthcoming books and news.

canopy-press.com | instagram.com/canopypress

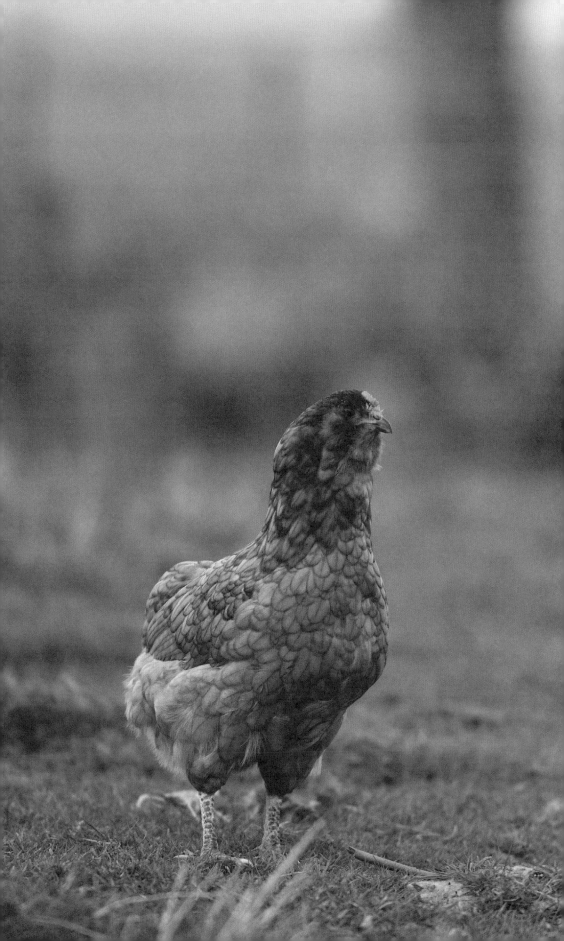

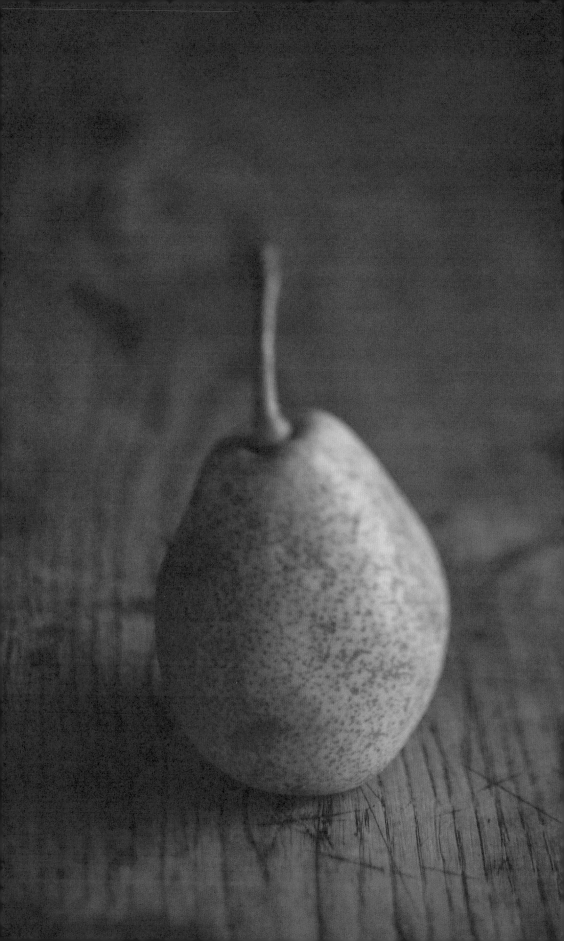

CONTENTS

FOREWORD

ROSIE BIRKETT

Food & cookery writer | instagram.com/rosiefoodie

It was my appetite that first got me into food, and it is hunger that has kept me here. As a child I was greedy, always buzzing around my mum – an exceptional home cook – as she prepared our family meals, on the scrounge for a scrap of whatever she could spare, be it a raw carrot baton, a corner of golden, flaky pastry (baked or raw, I wasn't fussy), or a sliver of roasted chicken skin.

At university, I would infuriate my housemates by hovering behind them as they cooked themselves student meals, asking questions about what exactly they were doing. In the office at my first magazine, I would lose my train of thought from whatever I was proofreading if I heard the rustle of a food packet; there were snacks inside my filing cabinet where there should have been stationery, and always a trail of incriminating crumbs around my desk. You get the idea. And so did my editor, who, probably in exasperation more than anything else, eventually set me loose on the Leeds restaurant scene as a restaurant reviewer. I have been writing about food and cookery ever since.

When I tell people I am a food and cookery writer, the response is often along the lines of: 'Does that mean you get to review restaurants and eat free food all the time?' And while I would be lying if I said that there isn't an element of that involved in what I do, and that it is a very nice perk of my job, these days my hunger takes a slightly different form. I am much more interested in exploring the roots of the food and drink we consume: the processes, personalities, and social and ethical implications of what we eat. Food is at once intensely personal and yet universal – it is anthropological, cultural, deeply complex, and rich with history and narrative. There is a story behind every mouthful, every crumb, every cup of morning tea or coffee, or glass of wine. It is these stories that fascinate and captivate me, and if you are reading this book, the chances are that you feel a similar curiosity.

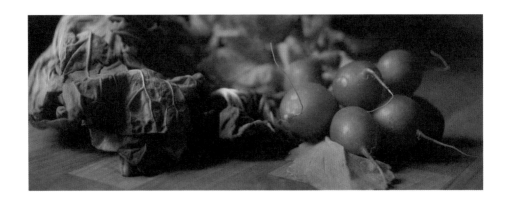

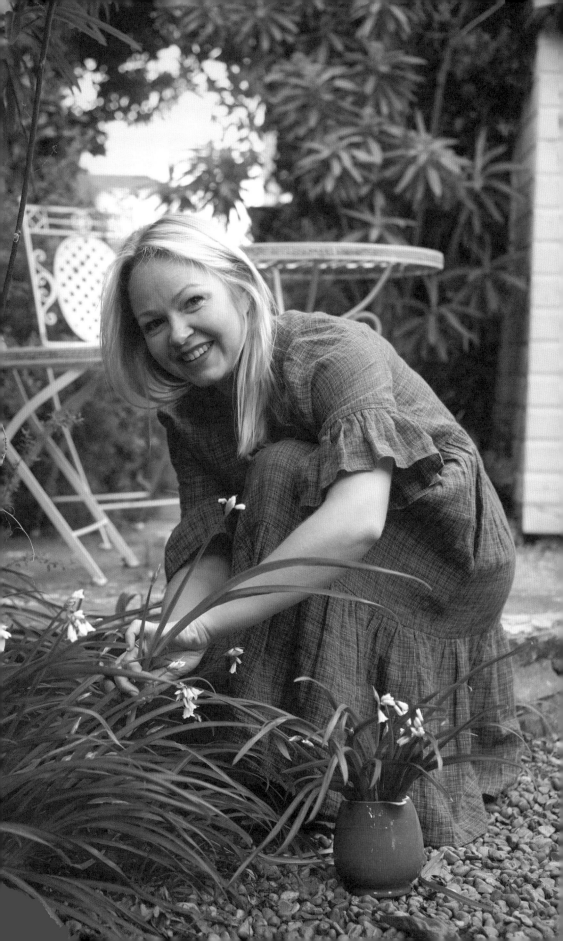

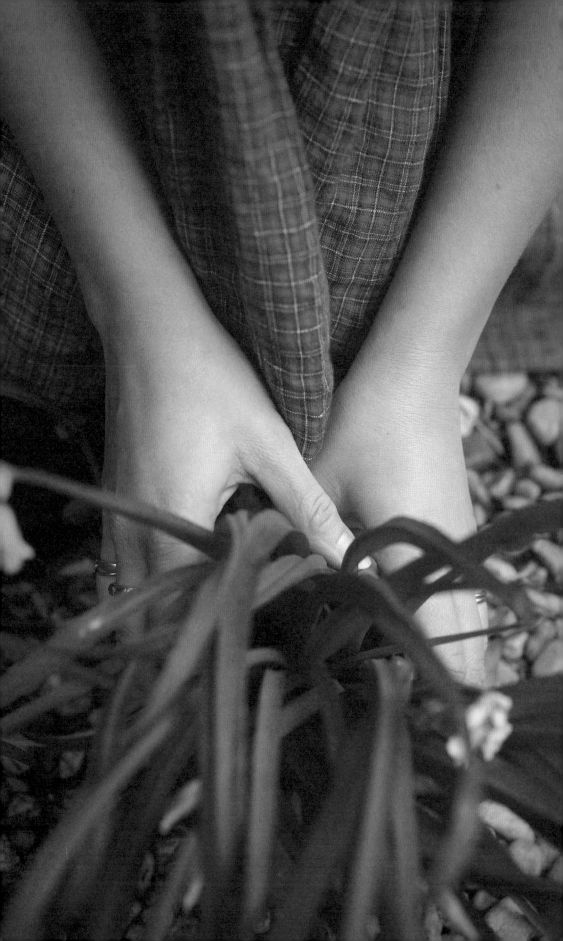

In terms of production, the global food system is far from perfect, with its reliance on imports and subsequent food miles, destructive agricultural practises promoting monocultures, and cheap, processed food that often depends on compromise at some level – whether ethically, environmentally, or in terms of workers' welfare – to keep costs down. But while the realities of feeding the world's growing population may seem bleak, there is also a slow and steady shift underway. Since I began my career over a decade ago, I have observed the common interest in the food and drink we purchase, cook, and consume surge. Among the general public – not just the people who consider themselves 'foodies' – there has been a heartening re-embracing of real, grass-roots food production methods, a penchant for provenance, and a new-found respect for the artisan.

"There is a yearning among consumers and producers, in domestic and professional kitchens alike, for a return to the tactile and sensory, and to the gratifyingly tangible craftsmanship of making"

A democratized culinary scene (the result of the last recession) and increased access to shareable knowledge, information, and ideas via the internet and social media, have resulted in a breaking down of some of the barriers around food and cookery. Whether it is having a go at a spot of preserving, fermenting, baking, or light foraging, people are skilling up and immersing themselves in both traditional and more innovative modes of production, with a strong emphasis on the craft of it all. In an increasingly mechanised and technological world, there is a yearning among consumers and producers, in domestic and professional kitchens alike, for a return to the tactile and sensory, and to the gratifyingly tangible craftsmanship of making.

For many of us, knowing where our food comes from and how it was produced has become an important part of our sense of well-being, and a lifestyle choice that can help us to feel more connected to our communities and the world we live in. At a moment in history when it is easy to feel lost amid the chaos, the small daily decisions we make, in terms of what we eat for breakfast, lunch, or dinner and put into our favourite mug or glass, can help us to feel that little bit more in control. Increasingly, in both small and large ways, people are turning away from industrialized, mass-produced products and looking to support their local and artisan producers or small-scale farmers.

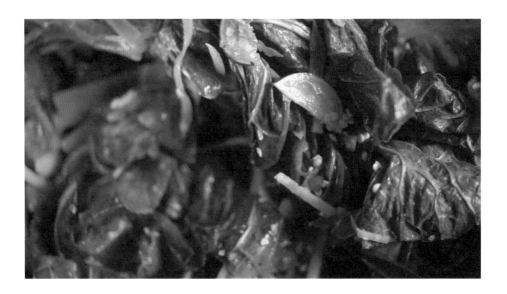

This book is a testament to that fact, and shines a light on a handful of brilliant people who represent a larger collective of passionate craftspeople throwing their energies and efforts into creating a more positive present and sustainable future for food. From the sourdough bakery renaissance to the natural wine movement, we are seeing a return to the honest, natural, agricultural values seemingly negated by the industrial food machine, and the bar is being raised for quality at every level.

It is now entirely possible to have as mind-blowing a plate of food for less than ten pounds at a street food van as it is from a tasting menu in a Michelin-starred restaurant. Likewise, when it comes to ingredients and staples we previously considered prosaic – whether coffee, chocolate, honey, wine, or bread – we are aware more now than ever that we can buy from a person, or small group of people, working hard and carefully to produce something not only of exceptional quality, but that expresses the uniqueness of its environment. We find wonderful examples of this in every chapter of *Gather & Nourish*: for example with Big Island Coffee Roasters, whose coffee trees are grown on a bed of lava and carry a particularly special minerality as a result, and with Bermondsey Street Bees, whose raw, unpasteurized honey boasts particularly complex and interesting flavours thanks to the array of forage available to its urban bees in London.

Gather & Nourish lifts the lid on these craftspeople, their passion, and the way they think, but also on how they make their businesses work on a practical level: how they make a living doing what they do. While it might sound romantic and whimsical to make a business from growing and roasting coffee in Hawaii, as Brandon and Kelleigh from Big Island Coffee very aptly put it: 'it's not all fairy tales and cupcakes.' This is a hard slog, especially when you are at the mercy of natural disasters and never sure when the next hurricane or volcano might hit, writing off your crop of ripe coffee cherries. The modern world can be a hostile place for food sustainability, and that is what makes these stories all the more inspiring. In the 'Honey' chapter, the people behind Bermondsey Street Bees explain the devastation that honeybees have faced because of monocultures and chemical industrial farming destroying the bees' habitat, and the diversity of the forage the bees need to survive and produce honey. I first met Dale and Sarah when I was filming a short film for *Saturday Kitchen*, and I remember being blown away by their knowledge, passion, and the restlessness they have to make a change on the landscape of global honey production. I remember thinking that they deserved much more airtime than the few minutes of our short, sharp film, and it is wonderful to read their story, told in their own words, and see it given the space it deserves.

As well as a dedication to quality and flavour, a common trope running through the profiles of the producers in this book is a strong sense of wider social responsibility, and being part of a much bigger picture, both in terms of food culture and community and the health and conservation of the planet. In her brilliantly powerful introduction, 'What Am I Eating?', writer and educator Jane Powell encourages us to think of ourselves as active food citizens, rather than passive consumers, whose choices can greatly improve and impact the world we live in, and by choosing to read this you are already making a difference. Savour every page, tell all the hungry people you know about it, buy it for like-minded and not-so-like-minded friends, and spread the word about the book that will nourish you with information, personal connection, and stories.

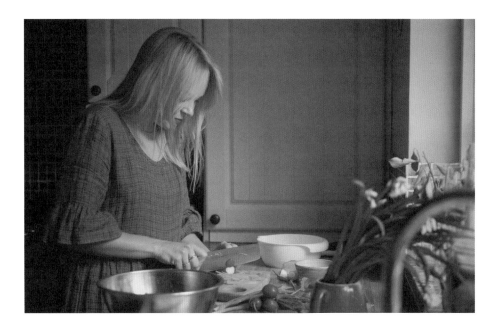

ABOUT THE AUTHOR

Rosie Birkett is a food and cookery writer with over a decade of experience in food media. Her books include *East London Food*, the critically acclaimed cookbook *A Lot on Her Plate*, and *The Joyful Home Cook*. Rosie is also a Soil Association and Fairtrade ambassador who aims to help improve the way people cook and eat. Visit rosiebirkett.com or find her on Instagram @rosiefoodie.

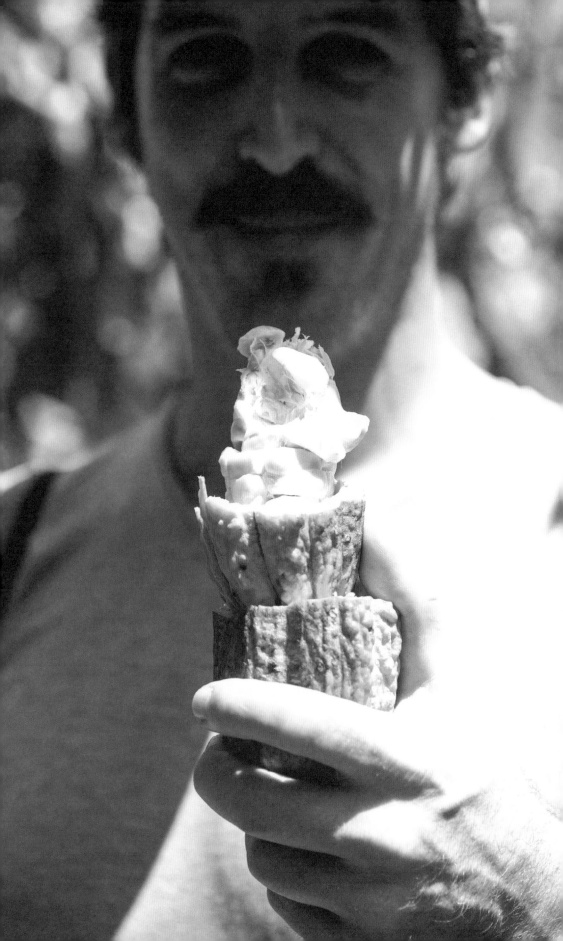

WHAT AM I EATING?

JANE POWELL

"Food is the supreme symbol of our
interconnectedness; the word 'companion'
means someone with whom we share bread
and suggests equality and respect"

THE INTRICACY OF FOOD

Food is complex. When you hold a piece of bread in your hand, you are connected not just to the farmer, miller, and baker who made it, but with humans thousands of years ago who domesticated wheat in the Middle East, and with generations since who have selected it for yield, flavour, and texture. You are also connected with the millions of microbes who populated the soil in which it grew, with the manufacturers of agricultural machinery, with lorry drivers, shop managers, supermarket shelf-stackers, packaging manufacturers, and food scientists. All these helped bring the loaf of bread to you.

You also share a connection with all the other people who are eating bread that came from the same baker, the same mill, the same field, or the same batch of seed. And, most obviously, you are connected with the people who share your table. Food is the supreme symbol of our interconnectedness; the word 'companion' means someone with whom we share bread and suggests equality and respect. It illustrates our dependence on each other and the natural world. Sun, rain, and soil feed all of us.

> "True mindfulness means gratitude to all those who helped to bring us the food, no matter how seemingly remote their connection"

It matters therefore what we eat, because it is a measure of how we care for each other, for the natural world, and for ourselves. It is important to eat healthily and to enjoy our food, but food is also about so much else. If we ourselves grow vegetables, bake bread or make blackberry jam for instance, we know the satisfaction of working with our hands and sharing food we have made with others, and it is natural to want the same fulfilment for others. So it matters how it's grown, processed, transported and traded. It makes a difference if it is made with care and attention by people who experience their work as an act of creative self-expression, and who receive a fair reward.

The growth of the Fairtrade label in recent years is a sign of how much better we feel eating food that has been produced under good conditions, from the field to our plates, and that we are willing to pay extra for that. We want growers and processors to be able to access education for their children, medical care and so on, and to be able to aspire to a more secure and rewarding life, just as we do ourselves. It is good to eat mindfully, but there is a lot more to that than simply being 'in the moment' with our sensual experience. True mindfulness means gratitude to all those who helped to bring us the food, no matter how seemingly remote their connection.

So what makes good food? In this book we will explore that question through the work of producers around the world who have faced that question and done their best to answer it. First, though, we need to look a bit more closely at the food chain. Where does food come from?

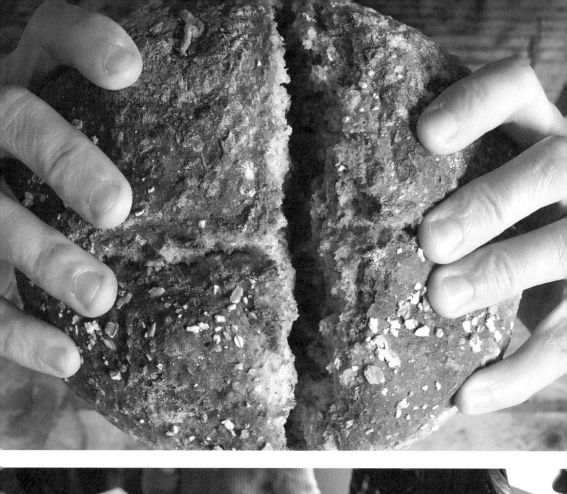
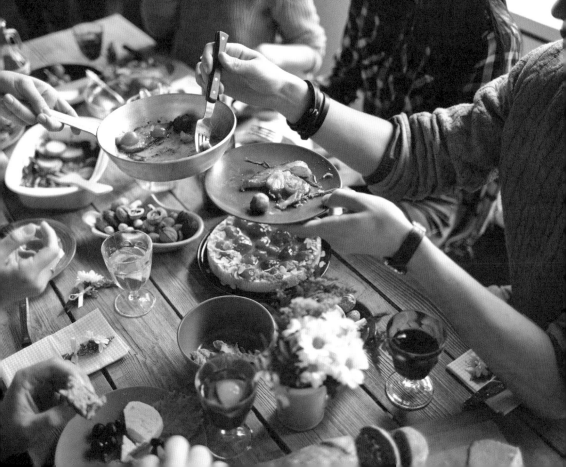

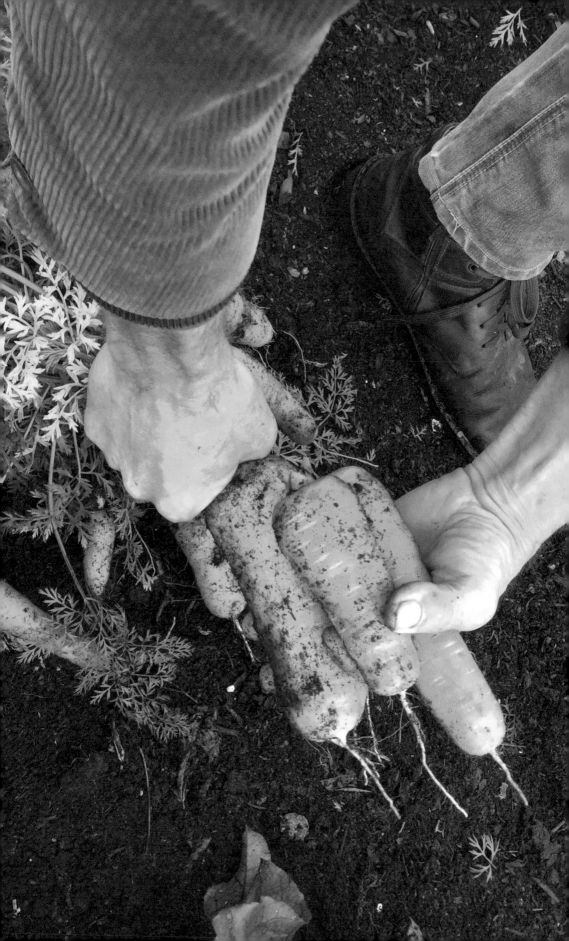

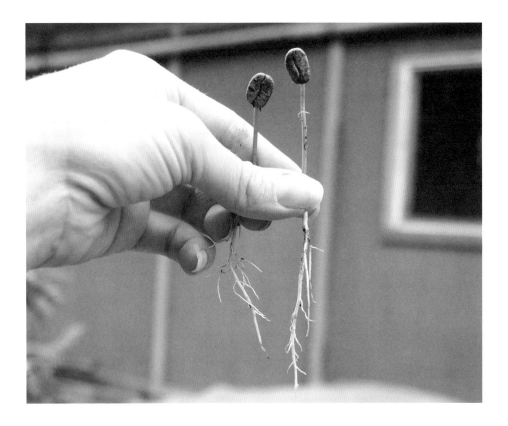

IT ALL STARTS WITH THE SOIL

Setting aside for a moment the food that is hunted or gathered from the wild – fish, seaweed, blackberries and so on – or cultured in artificial settings such as a laboratory or a soil-less greenhouse, most of what we eat comes from a farm or garden, and the story starts with the soil. We are accustomed to think of this as mud or dirt to be cleaned off our shoes or football kit, but it is a living and miraculous entity, and the health of the biosphere depends on it.

Soil forms where the earth's rocks are weathered into tiny particles by sun and rain, and it also hosts a huge range of bacteria, fungi, worms, and other creatures. These break down dead plants and animals and turn their remains into humus, the dark fibrous substance that holds water and nutrients and gives healthy soil its spongy, crumb-like consistency. That's why the biggest organic organization in the UK is called the Soil Association. Its founder, Lady Eve Balfour, was convinced that a healthy human population depended on a healthy soil, and she saw that the trend towards synthetic fertilizers and pesticides was disrupting that bond.

WHAT IS ORGANIC?

Organic farming is based on four principles:

ecology | care | health | fairness

The principle of ecology means farming that works with natural cycles, a concept also known as agroecology, or, in other words, ecology applied to agricultural systems. On farms, and also in your back garden, it means feeding the soil with compost or manure rather than supplying artificial fertilizer directly to the plant. It might mean protecting the soil from any cultivation that would disturb its structure and disrupt the biological processes that maintain fertility, as in 'no dig' gardening or minimum tillage farming. Crops are rotated, so that one year maybe you grow potatoes, which are heavy feeders, but the next year you grow beans to put nitrogen back in the soil, because all vegetables in the legume family, which includes beans, peas, and lentils, harbour nitrogen-fixing bacteria.

You can see this for yourself. Dig a clover plant out of your lawn and you will see small bead-like nodules on the roots. If you slice one in half with your fingernail, you will find it is pink inside because of a pigment that is closely related to the haemoglobin in our blood. We take oxygen out of the air and they take nitrogen.

Organic farming also means managing pests by various mechanical and biological means: for instance using resistant varieties, mixing crops in the same field, or encouraging natural predators by planting habitats for them. Arable farmers, for instance, may make a 'beetle bank', which is a grassy mound that runs through the middle of the crop. High standards of animal welfare allow livestock to express their natural behaviours, and the whole farm is managed so that birds, wildflowers, and invertebrates can flourish alongside food production as an integrated whole.

Linked to this, the principle of health is based on the concept of soil, plant, animal, and human making an indivisible whole that must be nurtured. Fairness refers to the human relationships of work and trade that interconnect with the biological processes of the farm, and care is about a precautionary and responsible approach to farming that takes future generations into account.

You can recognize organic food in a shop because it will say so on the packaging, which will also carry an organic certification number and probably the logo of one of the UK certification bodies, such as the Soil Association or Organic Farmers and Growers. It is important to state that the term 'organic' has a precise legal definition and it should not be used loosely just to mean 'unsprayed'. Organic farmers agree to abide by a detailed set of standards covering every aspect of the farm and are required to keep records, which are inspected annually. Processors such as bakers and manufacturers of ready meals can also sell their products as organic if they can prove that they have sourced their ingredients from organic farms and followed certain other rules. For instance, the food must not contain genetically modified organisms of any kind. Traders and importers are also certified.[1]

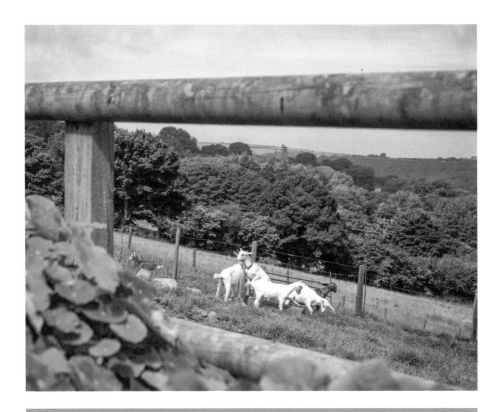

BIODYNAMICS

Biodynamic farming takes the organic principles a stage further by bringing in a spiritual dimension. It developed from a series of agricultural lectures given in 1924 by Austrian philosopher and social reformer Rudolf Steiner. Here the farm is seen as an organism in its own right, operating on a 'closed loop' that does not rely on feed or fertilizer brought in from outside. As in organic farming, with which it shares very similar standards, compost is essential to maintaining soil fertility. However, on biodynamic farms there is a special role for cow manure, which may be added to the compost in very small quantities, and there is a requirement to use highly diluted medicinal plant preparations in order to activate the microbes that are fundamental to the process. In addition, many biodynamic farmers follow a calendar for planting, sowing, and harvesting that is based on lunar and planetary movements.

These practices all reflect the belief that the farm is receiving and mediating cosmic energies that go beyond those understood by conventional agricultural science. This is not a view everyone will share, but biodynamic farming has been extensively tried and tested by its practitioners and there is some scientific evidence for its effectiveness in maintaining soil fertility.[2]

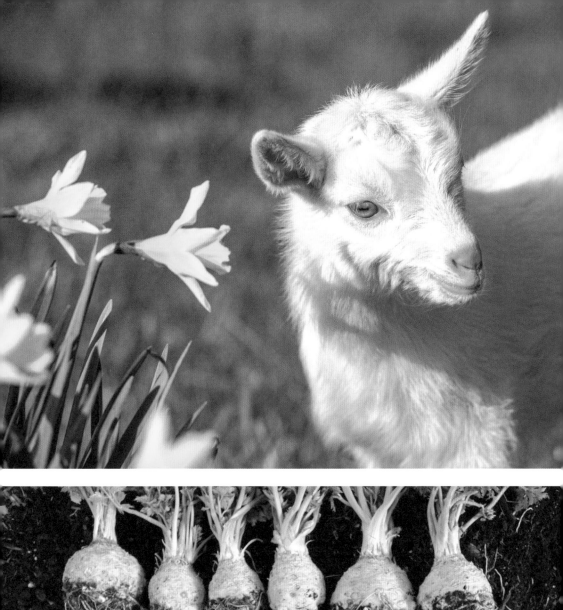

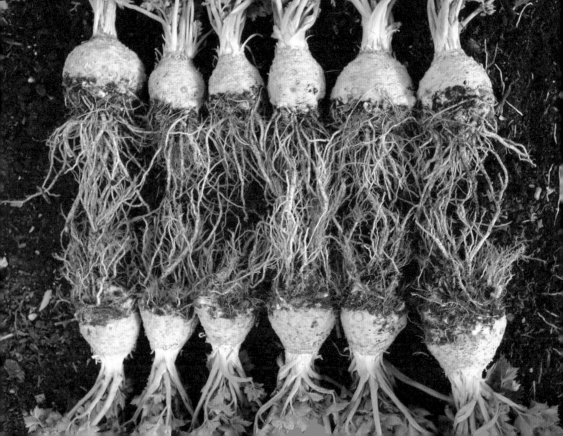

THE INEVITABILITY OF COMPROMISE

The organic certification system is not perfect, of course. There are areas where the vision of natural perfection meets the real world and compromises are made. For instance, although organic farmers take a preventative approach to animal health, livestock must be given antibiotics or other drugs if they need them for the sake of their welfare. To manage this, a withdrawal period is set to allow the drug to leave their system before they become food. If bad weather causes a severe shortage of fodder, organic farmers may obtain permission from their certifying body to buy in non-organic silage or hay.

Organic farming does not have a monopoly on good food production: there are many excellent examples of so-called conventional farming that may be informed by generations of good practice. Often small farmers and growers do not seek organic certification because their businesses are too small to justify the sheer cost of the annual inspection or because they prefer to rely on their own local reputation, being accountable to their customers. Many food producers and makers may follow broadly agroecological principles but make pragmatic adjustments that do not follow the letter of organic farming. Where there is no relationship between producer and customer however, certification provides a vital element of trust.

There are other farming certification systems too. In the UK, for instance, the LEAF Marque (LEAF means Linking Environment And Farming) recognizes a system of Integrated Farm Management, which covers such elements as energy efficiency, pollution control, and community engagement while allowing judicious use of agrochemicals. RSPCA Assured is a farm animal welfare scheme that includes space for the animals, natural lighting, and an enriched environment, allowing animals to express natural behaviours, including play.

Marine Stewardship Council certification covers seafood, Fairtrade is about fair prices and working conditions for farmers in developing countries, and Pasture for Life means that sheep and cows have been reared exclusively on grass and forage crops. All of these labels show that the producer has taken steps to improve their methods; taken together they help to build trust and accountability in the food system. Some of the certifying bodies, such as the Fairtrade Foundation, work internationally. Others, such as the organic ones, only inspect UK producers and processors, but a system of equivalence agreements with other countries means that they can certify imported products and be confident that their supply chains follow the same standards.

None of them are perfect, because good farming and food preparation involve so many factors and it is impossible to optimize the system for all. Is our priority animal welfare, or wildlife, or personal health, or global justice? These, and others, are aspects of good food that we each need to weigh up for ourselves.

MAKING

Most of the food we eat is not raw, straight from nature. It is usually cooked or processed in some way, to preserve it, to improve the flavour, or to destroy toxins. Often these treatments involve microbial processes that have been developing over millennia and which result in a richly complex food that carries within it the history of a local area. This is true, for instance, of a cheese that has absorbed bacteria from the pasture of the farm where the cow grazed, or a natural wine that contains its own unique blend of yeasts.

> "[Processing methods] represent skills
> which may take a lifetime to perfect
> and which are an expression of cultural
> identity that enriches our lives"

Fermenting is a technology that has been passed from person to person throughout history and is freely available to us now in the democratic way of microbes. You can create your own sourdough culture by leaving a bowl of flour and water out for a few days in your kitchen and it will be uniquely yours. Or you can make sauerkraut from cabbage and salt and be part of an age-old tradition of preserving vegetables for long European winters.

Other processing methods include drying, smoking, salting, and, of course, cooking. They represent skills which may take a lifetime to perfect and which are an expression of cultural identity that enriches our lives. They provide meaningful and satisfying work and result in food that nourishes our minds and imaginations as well as our bodies. They can be an expression of local culture in the same way that a language is: think of Iberico ham from pigs grazed under oak trees in the *dehesa* of Spain, or Stilton cheese from the rich pasturelands of England's East Midlands, or hummus made from chickpeas domesticated in the eastern Mediterranean millennia ago.

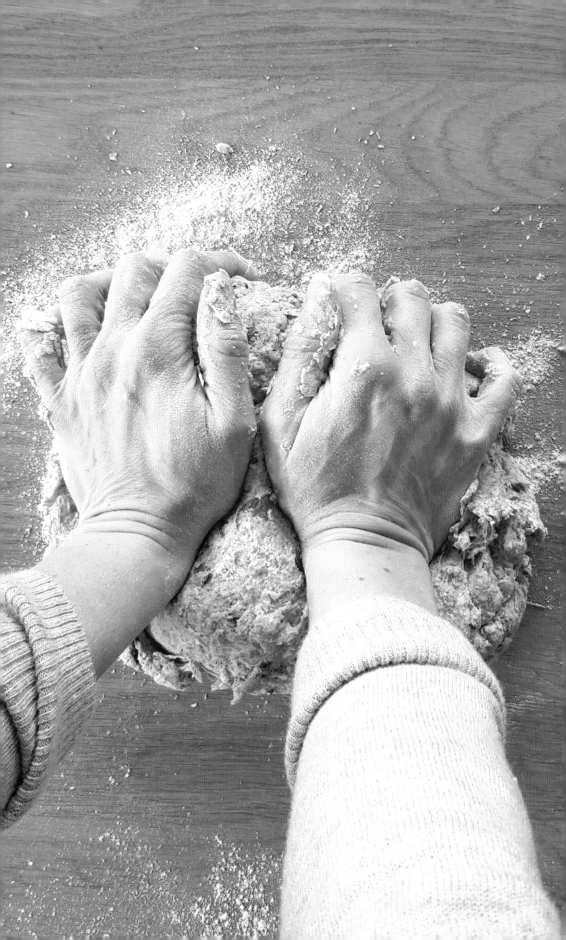

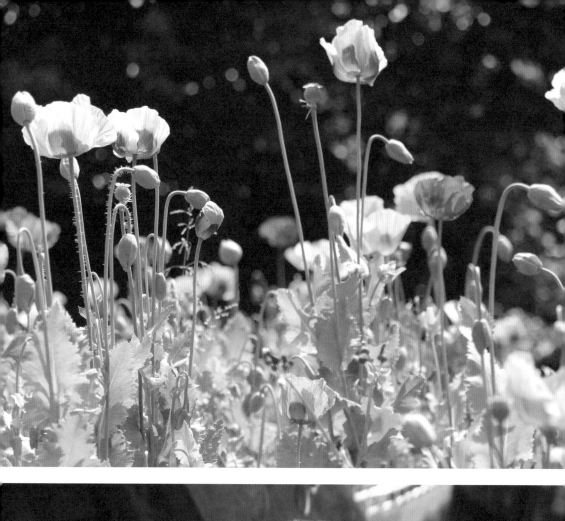

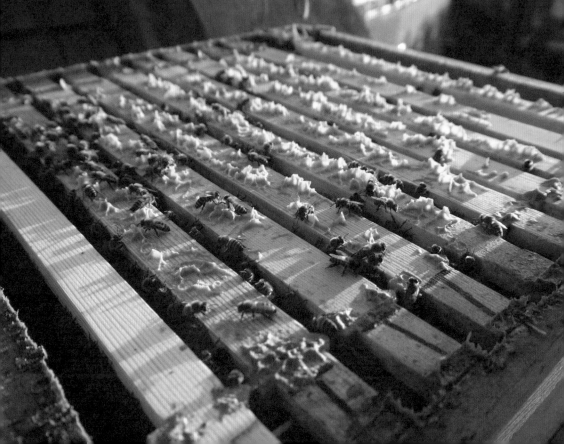

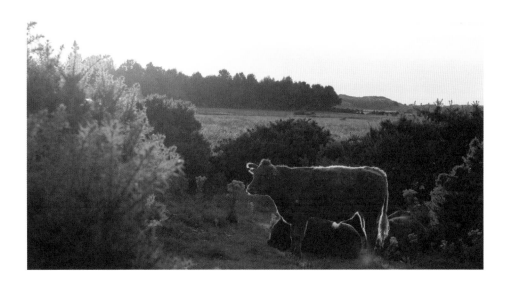

WHAT ARE THE REAL COSTS?

Any discussion of good food sooner or later comes up against the question of money. This is often asked rhetorically – *who is going to pay that much for a loaf of bread?* – as if to imply that food should by right be cheap. That is the thinking implied by the term 'food poverty', as if the excessive cost of food is the reason some go without. By this logic the expensive artisan loaf is elitist, while the supermarket ready-sliced version is more democratic and egalitarian, not to say thrifty. But such moral judgments obscure the really important questions that lie behind the cost of food.

The deeper question is this: what sort of food system do we want, and how can we use our purchasing power to create that? For money should be in service to a healthy and fair food system, and it should not call the shots. This is a big mental step to take. In our industrialized society, where traditional communities have weakened and we live as if the natural world were a force that we have conquered, money has come to have a powerful emotional significance. Taking a closer look at how we spend it, and where we place food in our list of priorities, can be uncomfortable.

> "The deeper question is this: what sort of food system do we want, and how can we use our purchasing power to create that?"

But there is no reason for guilt here. We absorb the values of the society around us until we start to question them, and once we do, we are free to come into a more empowered relationship with money. So how do we marry up this system of abstract and impersonal accounting called money, with a food system that expresses our values of care, human relationships, and balance with nature?

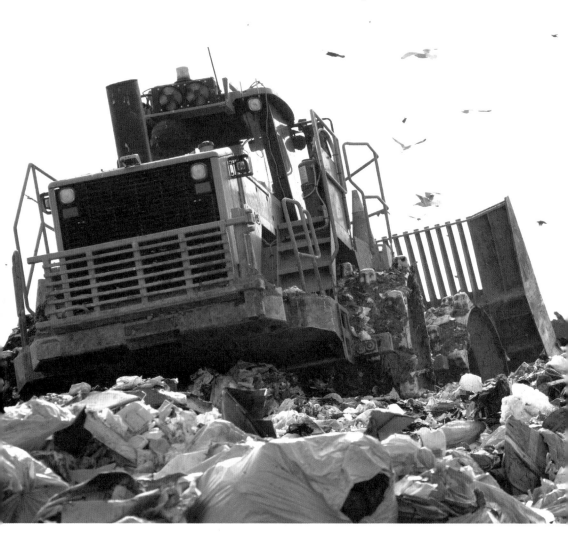

A CHANGE IN THINKING

The main point to grasp is that 'cheap food' is not really cheap at all. If you add back into the cost of your weekly shop all the other expenses associated with making it, the bill goes up. It's just that you won't be paying it at the till: you will pay it through your taxes and insurance, or your children will, or maybe people in other countries will carry the burden. Someone has to clean up the water supply that is polluted when nitrate fertilizer runs off the field into the river.

Someone also has to pay the medical costs of dealing with the epidemic of diabetes and obesity, which is strongly linked to poor diets. When yields drop as a result of soil erosion, or because the bees are in decline, or because of climate change caused in part by an energy-guzzling food system, then again, it has a cost. What is needed is a way of putting these factors back into the equation by a system of true cost accounting, such as the one advocated by the Sustainable Food Trust. Meanwhile, we can all bear these insights in mind when we decide how much we want to pay for good food.

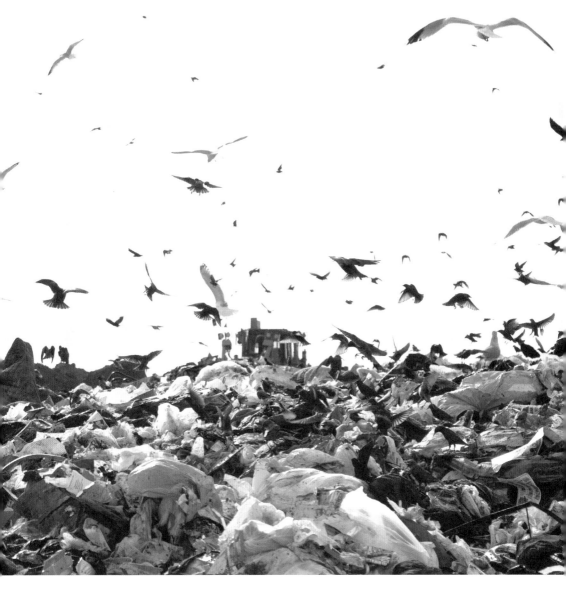

An example that is easy to relate to is the shocking extent of food waste. The fact that some thirty to fifty per cent of food grown on farms never makes it to our stomachs shows how crazy our relationship with money has become. In financial terms, it makes some sort of sense for food supply chains to run at high levels of waste in order to provide 'the consumer' with just the right sort of cosmetically perfect product we have come to expect, and to ensure the shelves are always well-stocked so that they don't wander off to another shop instead.

But in real terms, how can it be right to waste so much food, and all the labour, time, and resources that went into growing and making it? It is a sign of the gap that has developed between money and the real world, and we can start to mend it by using food wisely at home. We can make shopping lists so we don't buy too much on impulse, and find creative uses for leftovers.

WHAT CAN WE DO?

It is time to assign food its proper value and to be prepared to pay a little extra premium for food that has been produced in ways that seem good to us. Rather than resenting the extra cost, we can see it as an investment in the natural world, in soil health and in the dignity of human labour and culture. Together we can build a new food system based on the values that we want to see, and in so doing we reclaim our agency and power.

This means understanding our food better. It's only good to pay a high price for food if we know it to be aligned with the values we care about. All too often, we pay a premium for sophisticated packaging, convenience, celebrity endorsement or a clever marketing campaign. We need to have our wits about us; we need to move beyond 'consumer choice' and start exercising the responsibilities of a citizen. This means choosing food that gives us pleasure not just because it tastes good but also because we know it was produced in a way that honours the connections between 'plate, planet, people, politics, and culture', as the Slow Food Movement puts it.[3]

Meanwhile, although it costs to produce good food, there are ways of bringing food bills back down. Eating seasonally and buying fresh ingredients is one; the UK strawberry season is already several months long – maybe we don't need them in December. Highly processed foods like crisps, ready meals and fizzy drinks could be an occasional treat rather than a store cupboard staple. Meat, too, is a good example of a product where it makes sense to buy less often but spend more, for the sake of animal welfare and environmental benefits.

Nose-to-tail eating, which means eating offal such as liver and tripe, makes full use of an animal's carcass and also keeps a traditional food culture alive, as well as saving money. And of course plant-based eating tends to be cheaper.

Buying from local shops and farmers' markets where you can talk to the grower or maker and find out what they do is another way to get the most benefit out of our food spending. This has the added advantage that your money stays in the local economy, where it circulates and benefits other businesses, rather than being sucked out by a supermarket's head office and passed to shareholders.

COMMUNITY SUPPORTED AGRICULTURE

For the intrepid food citizen, there are Community Supported Agriculture schemes where you can pay upfront for a season's produce and share the risks of production. Typically these revolve around fruit and vegetables, but there are also micro-dairies providing goats' and cows' milk, and livestock farms supplying meat boxes. There are many variations on the theme of direct sales, including food hubs and food assemblies, which allow for flexibility but still give the customer a direct link with the producer in a relationship that is enriching for both sides.

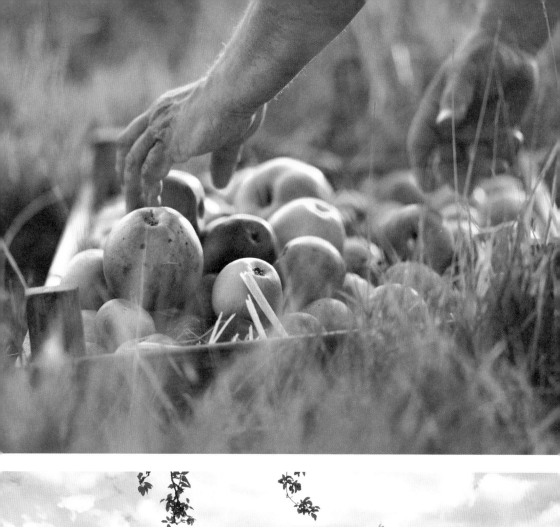

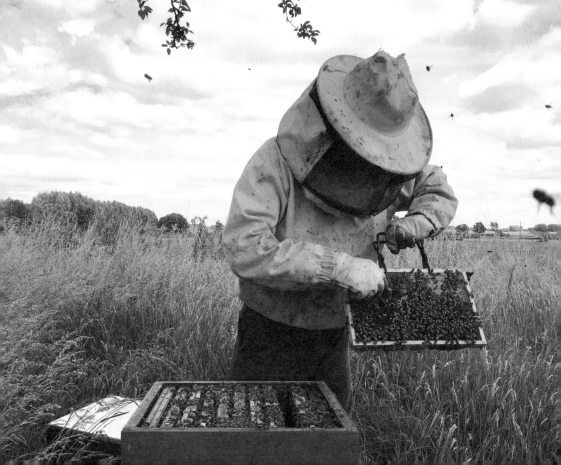

GOOD FOOD IS FOR EVERYBODY

Ecologically and nutritionally sound food chains are not enough if they come with unrewarding, low-paid jobs – another reason to question cheap food. A food system based on compassionate values should honour the dignity of human labour, and indeed there are many food businesses that make this their *raison d'être*. There are community bakeries that provide placements for people with mental health problems, urban gardens that tackle youth unemployment, and restaurants that train prisoners for a new career.

Other food businesses, run along more commercial lines, may still be inspiring places for creative expression and allow people to gain satisfaction from using their skills to benefit others, while paying a fair wage. They may also make a valuable contribution to the communities in which they live through sponsorship, education or events. Good food is for everybody.

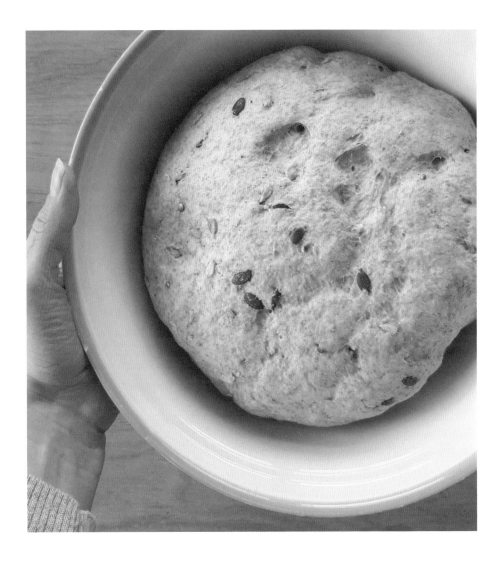

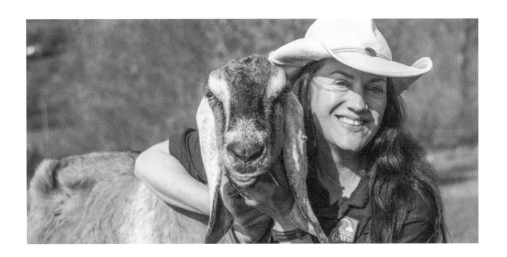

BECOMING A FOOD CITIZEN

Educate yourself about the food you eat.

Read labels and buy food that matches your values.

Grow and make some food yourself, so you understand it with your body and not just your mind.

Look around your local community and ask yourself what sort of food culture it has. Who is producing food? Does everyone have enough to eat? Consider volunteering for a community garden or surplus-food distribution project.

Lobby politicians for better food for all.

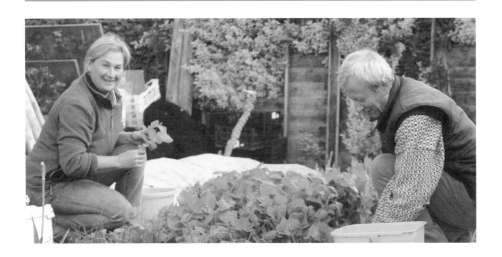

THE FUTURE

We have a more globalized food system than ever before. This means that we can, if we make the effort, enjoy a highly varied diet that is not only nutritionally sound but also enriches our lives culturally. And yet for many people, food means a narrow set of variations on a highly processed theme, high in calories, salt, and sugar, and low on nutrients. Meanwhile, our intricate global trading system makes us very vulnerable to disruptions. Food is delivered to supermarkets on a just-in-time basis, which means that there is limited warehouse storage to tide us over disruptions – even bad weather can cause temporary shortages. And, of course, the increasing unpredictability of our climate makes us vulnerable to droughts, floods, and freezes around the world.

There is talk again of food security, a term that has long been out of fashion, and calls for fresh thinking. Do we want to see a food system that is more local, meeting human needs for belonging and a sense of place as well as buffering us against global forces? Do we want to support a food system that provides more rewarding employment in our communities and allows people to reconnect with nature? Do we want our food to be made by people who find satisfaction in developing their skills and feel they have some control over their lives? These are questions that will be decided by all of us as we decide where to spend our food budgets, and which politicians to vote for.

> "We can, if we make the effort, enjoy a highly varied diet that is not only nutritionally sound but also enriches our lives culturally"

We have discussed the general principles of food production and manufacture and looked at some of the criteria that we might use in deciding what to buy and eat. But it is really only through learning about the details of particular businesses that the principles come to life. What does growing and processing food really look like? What does it feel like? What are the joys and the challenges?

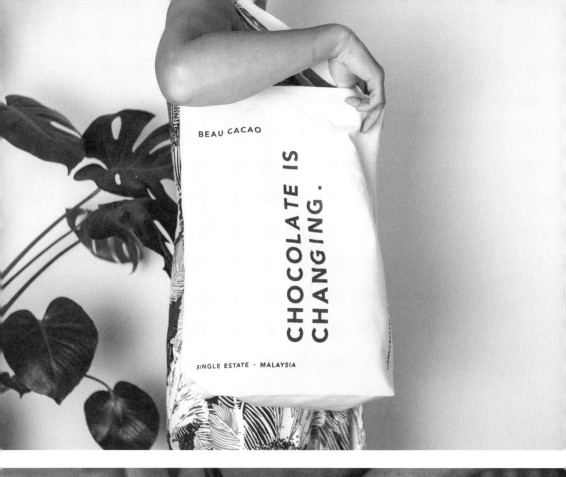

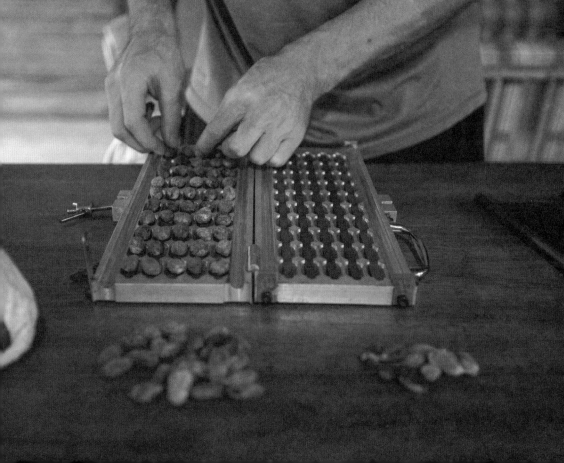

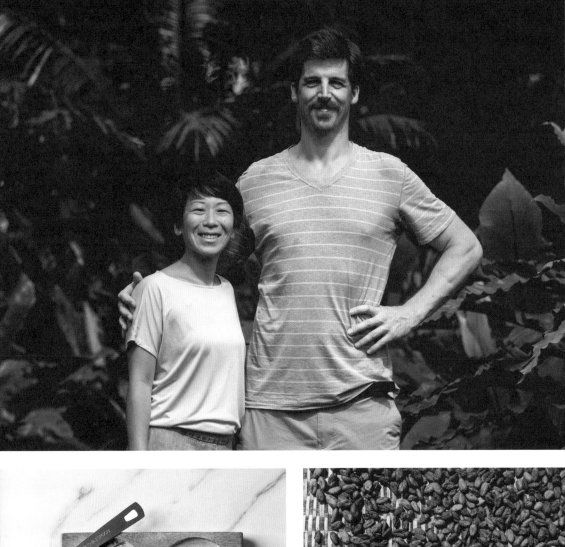

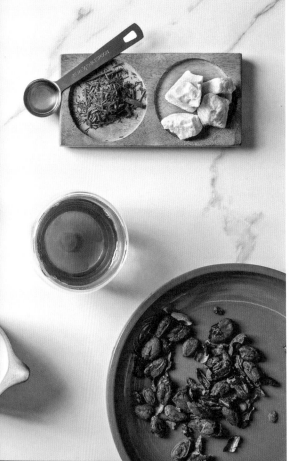

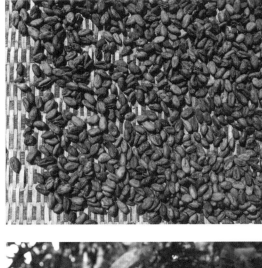

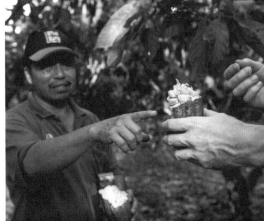

A STARTING POINT

In this book we will meet a number of enterprises that are producing food in the best way they know how. These are people who have followed their passions – and it takes a lot of passion to get you through the hard grind of starting and running a small business. They are real people in real situations, and none of them are perfect. It is probably true to say that most of them didn't set out to be, either.

All of them must grapple with the contradictions of our modern society, where things that would do us good in the long term, like healthy food and wildlife-friendly farming, are seen as unaffordable in the short term. That can make it hard for an ecologically sound food business to keep afloat unless they are producing a luxury or niche product, for which they can charge a higher price, and are prepared to work very hard. Add to that the proliferation of regulations intended to bring us safer food – such as the requirement to have a vet in attendance at an abattoir, or to pasteurize milk – and the practical considerations that mean it is hard to avoid wrapping food in plastic or transporting it in diesel vans, and there is no such thing as a perfectly sustainable food business.

Some pioneering companies are featured in this book, and we hope that they will inspire you to look for more where you live. They are often run at a human scale, meeting the particular needs of a particular locality and responding to opportunities that have come up. No two are the same, but they do all share some common values. They are about human skill and artistry, and they centre on a personal approach. Many of them are organic, and others stand for agroecological principles. In their different ways, they pick up the strands of tradition and make something new out of them.

"There is no such thing as a perfectly sustainable food business"

CONSUMERS OR CITIZENS?

No discussion of the food system would be complete without mention of the all-important 'consumer' for whose benefit this intricate web of relationships has been constructed. The purpose of this book is to dismantle the idea that we are passive individuals whose only function is to spend and support the economy. Here we present a bigger picture of what is possible. By looking behind the scenes of the food world and gaining an insight into the joys and dilemmas that come with feeding people, the hope is that we will encourage you to buy food responsibly, creatively, and intelligently.

Not only that, but you might like to try your own hand at some of the food-making methods described here. Gardening, baking bread, fermenting vegetables, making jam, and brewing beer were originally small-scale domestic activities, and they still can be. They can be satisfying and empowering in their own right, and they can readily be extended to make microbusinesses. You could find yourself selling your produce at a farmers' market or school fete, or bartering with your neighbours. And you just might find that you have the makings of a full-time livelihood.

We may feel powerless in the face of the large corporations that control much of the food system, but we need to remember that we have agency too. The small businesses in these pages reveal the basics of food production and show an alternative. By buying from them and others like them, and not only that, enquiring further into what they do, visiting them, and giving them feedback, we move out of the helplessness of the consumer. We begin to see ourselves as food citizens, helping to shape the future of food.

FURTHER READING

FOOD CITIZENSHIP foodcitizenship.info

TRUE COST ACCOUNTING Sustainable Food Trust. 'The True Cost of Food.'
Available at sustainablefoodtrust.org/key-issues/true-cost-accounting

FOOD WASTE Stuart, Tristram. *Waste: Uncovering the Global Food Scandal.* London: Penguin, 2009.

ABOUT THE AUTHOR

Jane Powell is an independent writer, editor, and activist based in Wales. She has worked in agricultural science publishing, as a teacher, as Project Officer with Organic Centre Wales in 2000–2015, and as Education Coordinator with LEAF (Linking Environment And Farming) Education since 2006. Visit foodsociety.wales.

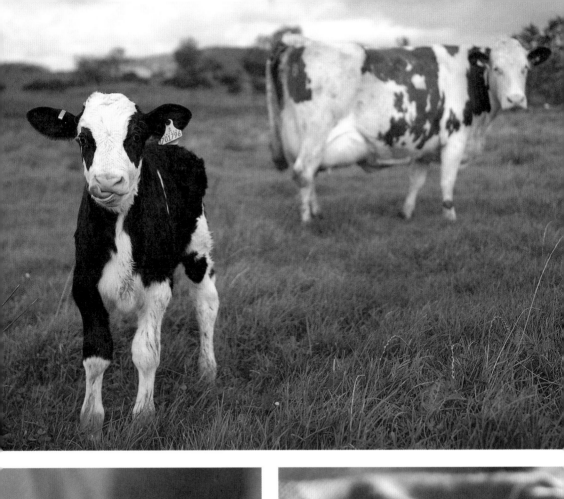

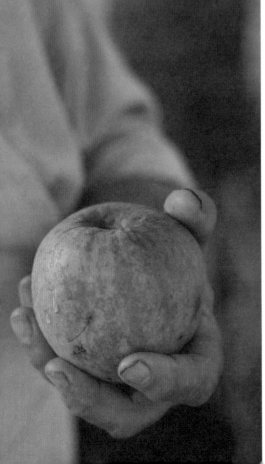

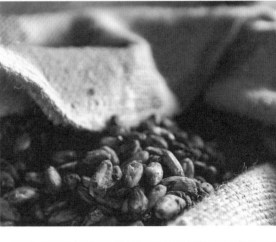

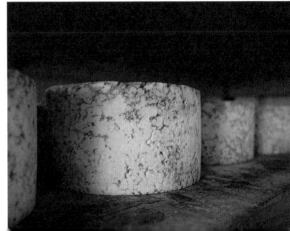

BIODIVERSITY

Biodiversity is the variety of life on earth, from microscopic organisms to whole ecosystems. We as a species are reliant on biodiversity to survive – for example, if we didn't have bees then fruit-bearing plants wouldn't be pollinated, and we would have no fruit. For this reason, biodiversity loss is a significant threat to the planet and everything living on it. As the human population increases, so does the pressure on biodiversity, from the extinction of animals through unsustainable hunting to the loss of important habitat and plantation due to the expansion of farmland. Protecting and celebrating biodiversity is therefore something we can take into account when trying to make more sustainable food choices.

In this section we will look at how a range of different producers consider biodiversity as part of their business ethos. The Ethical Dairy chapter will focus not on cheese but dairy farming, going back to the source to explore ways ecological farming can have a positive impact on the biodiversity crisis. 'Closing the loop', protecting species, and maintaining health will be key themes across these chapters as we then delve into the delectable world of kefir, honey, and apple cider vinegar.

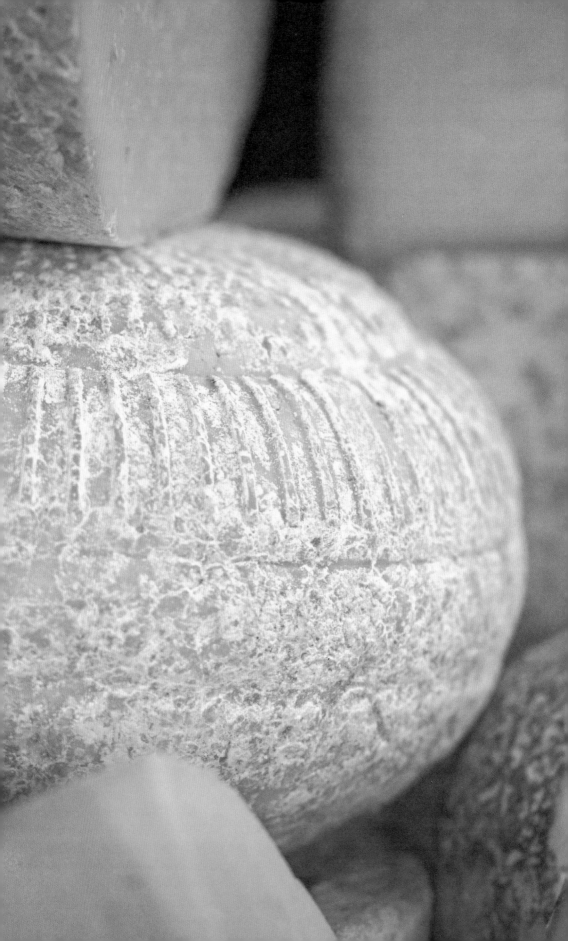

CHEESE

Cheese is an ancient food that is valued across the world as being rich in proteins, fats, and calcium. It is mostly made from cows' milk but can be made from the milk of sheep, goats, buffalo, yaks, camels, and reindeer. It is likely to have been discovered accidentally, thousands of years ago, when milk was transported in pouches made from sheeps' stomachs, and the rennet in the pouches separated the milk into curds and whey. It has come a long way since those early days and there are now thousands of varieties globally.

"We have a closed-loop bacterial cycle, producing a cheese that is unique to that farm. That is the concept behind the old description of a cheese's 'terroir'"

David Finlay, The Ethical Dairy

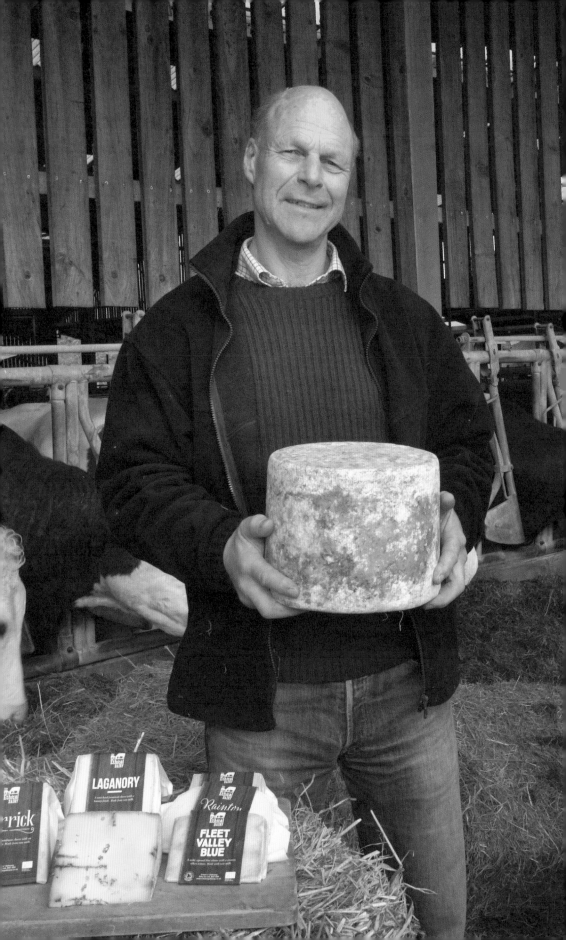

THE ETHICAL DAIRY

DAVID FINLAY

Castle Douglas, Scotland | theethicaldairy.co.uk

I took over the family farm, Rainton, in 1987, tenanting 850 acres of fairly remote, rugged, coastal upland with dairy, beef, and sheep. Our family has farmed almost continuously in this area for the past couple of hundred years. Before I returned to the farm I was working as a farm advisory consultant. At that time I was very dismissive of organic or any ecological farming – like many in the 1980s I considered it a joke, a waste of money and resources. Once I was actually working on the farm, however, I found I wasn't comfortable with the pressure I felt to intensify. I grew disillusioned with the spiralling costs and mortality of the stock, and uncomfortable with the amount of chemicals we were applying to land and stock. Stocking levels were up, we were more and more dependent on feed and fertilizers, and as a consequence morbidity was up, mortality was up, and so was antibiotic usage.

I wanted to try something different. My sister has an organic smallholding and Wilma, my wife, was interested in all things organic. In the late 1990s organic products were becoming popular and the time seemed right to try it. Ten years later we were committed, and had familiarized ourselves with the practices of organic farming.

During this time we had started to open our farm up to members of the public, with farm tours running daily through our ice cream visitor attraction, Cream o' Galloway. We started to see our farm through the eyes of our visitors, from a non-farming point of view. We found that one of the most frequently asked questions was: 'Why do you separate the calves from the cows?' This practice is standard in dairy farming to allow the milk to be extracted from the mother as soon as possible, with none spared for the calf. As a result, the calves don't receive the nutritional or emotional benefits of their mother's milk. This prompted us to ask ourselves: 'What would happen if we didn't separate the calves from their mothers?'

RETHINKING THE FARMING SYSTEM

Rainton Farm was generally well-known as a dairy farm that made traditional farmhouse cheddar. In fact, cheese was still being made here as recently as the 1970s before large-scale cheddar manufacturing led to the closure of our local small-scale cheese production. We took a few years to relearn the craft of traditional cheese-making and we formally launched our new cheeses under the brand The Ethical Dairy in 2018.

Why do we claim to be ethical? Well, the main difference between us and many other dairy farms in the country is that for the past decade we have been working towards developing a system of cow-with-calf dairy farming that is viable and sustainable at scale. It has not been easy. We have had to build a new dairy that could accommodate the calves alongside their mothers, and have had to completely rethink how we manage the herd. We had an unsuccessful pilot in 2013 that failed spectacularly but which taught us a great deal. As of 2019 we are three years into a full roll-out of cow-with-calf dairy farming and we can now say with some confidence that our system is working.

We take less milk from the cows than a conventional dairy farm but we use that milk to produce ice cream and artisan cheese. By turning our fresh milk into food products we should eventually be able to remove our reliance on wholesale milk markets and make our business more resilient. Using the milk on site to create our own products also creates more jobs, which helps to sustain our local rural economy. We are driven by the belief that by rethinking the farming industry, we can produce nutritious food and comfortably feed our population without destroying the environment. We want to prove that an ecological approach to food production, one that works with natural systems rather than against them, is the solution to the challenges facing our industry, our health, and our planet.

"Our cows live unusually long, productive lives where they are able to express natural behaviour in a landscape that benefits from their grazing"

We are therefore trying to create a food producing system that is sustainable in the long term without causing harm to the planet. We are doing that by moving towards an almost closed-loop (waste-free) system where we have enough animals to be sustained on pasture from the farm, producing waste that we turn into energy and digestate, which is then used to rejuvenate the soil. We have also carried out other environmental improvements, such as developing ponds designed for insects and planting broad-leaved trees for red squirrels. Since our farm is less intensive, our cows live unusually long, productive lives where they are able to express natural behaviour in a landscape that benefits from their grazing.

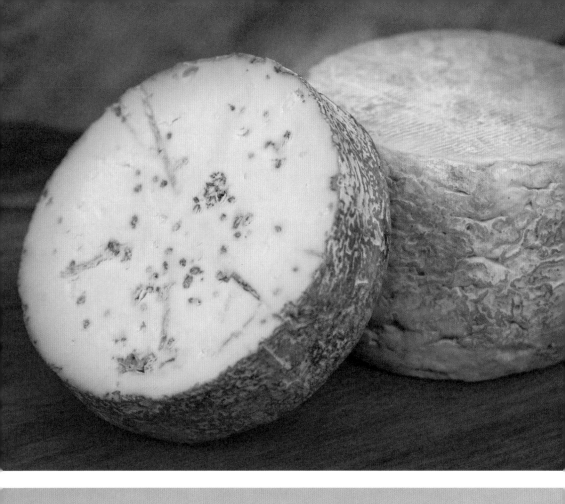

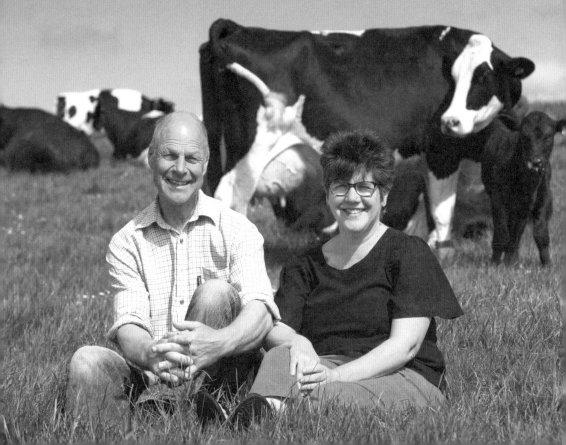

HOW DO WE WORK?

Grass On our farm we grow grass. It is just about the only crop that will grow on our farm. While humans can't eat grass, ruminant animals do. Those animals then produce high-quality dairy and nutritious red meat. We are a 'Pasture for Life' farm, which means that we do not feed our animals any form of grain or manufactured feeds.

Grazing Through grazing the grass our cattle rejuvenate the soil, adding natural fertilizer and locking carbon into the soil. The grazing action of the cattle compacts the soil and replicates the actions of the large herds of grazing animals that used to roam the grasslands of the world. This activity rebuilds our soil biome, locks carbon into the soil, and reduces the risk of surface water run-off with its inherent soil erosion and flooding consequences. This is now known as 'regenerative farming' and is being seen as a critical component of a sustainable food system.

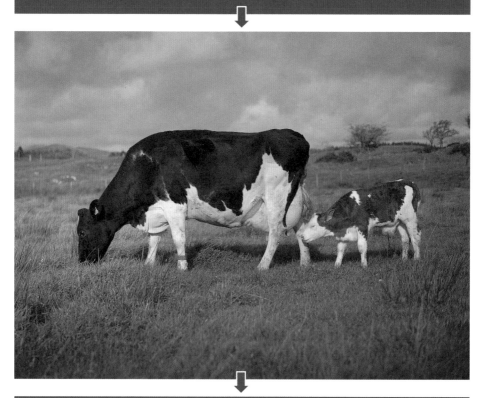

Milk Our herd produces high-quality milk. We milk the cows only once a day, in the morning. For the remainder of the day the calves get to stay with their mum to suckle. This results in the calves thriving, growing much faster than conventional dairy calves, which means that the heifers (females) join the dairy herd earlier than on conventional farms, while the bullocks (males) enter the meat trade to produce very high-quality young beef.

Cheese The milk is used to create both ice cream and cheese. The cheese is made in small batches using traditional processes to create high-quality artisan cheeses. These are slowly matured for up to eighteen months. We sell the cheese direct via our website and through wholesalers and retailers.

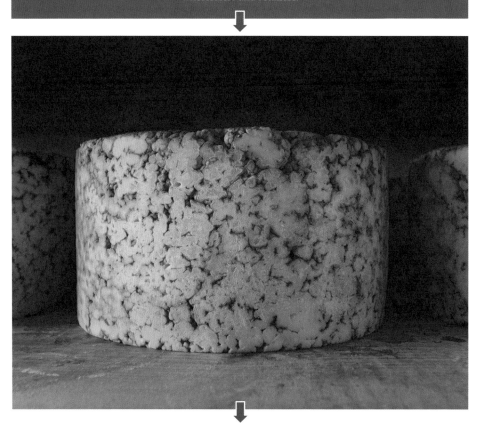

Packaging As far as possible we use sustainable materials in our packaging, including recycled paper and 'woolcool' to regulate mail-order pack temperatures. Unfortunately, we have yet to find an alternative to plastic for our cheese packaging. Plastic helps to prolong the shelf life and maintain product quality, but we are hopeful that customer demand in the industry generally will result in more sustainable packaging being developed.

Waste Our slurry and farm waste goes into our purpose-built anaerobic digester, which creates energy to power our cheese dairy and our hot water. The digestate, effectively a liquid compost, that is left over is used on our pasture because it is a more effective fertilizer and much kinder to our natural environment than raw slurry, which is what is traditionally used on dairy farms.

THE FARMING DEBATE

To understand why The Ethical Dairy's farming and food production system is so unusual, you need to appreciate how intensified conventional farming has become, and consequently the damage it does to the environment, the animals, and the people who work within that intensive system. The resulting negative outcomes include antibiotic resistance, poor animal welfare, social deprivation, biodiversity loss, diffuse pollution, greenhouse gas emissions, and resource depletion.

The main beneficiaries of our current food production system assert that more of the same is our best option to sustainably feed our planet, and that any shortfalls of our current food system can be overcome by the development and application of existing and future technologies. They also suggest that by increasing production from this food model – intensification – the negative side-effects of this approach can be diluted over more kilos or litres. Thus the 'per unit of food produced' impact on our lives and world is less, while jobs and growth are generated in our high-tech sector.

At the other end of the scale, there are those that contend that farming animals for food is unethical, damaging to our health and environment, and is a major contributor to global food insecurity. They propose that land released from livestock production could be rewilded, producing additional environmental benefits. This is a powerful argument, and one that would also involve major social, economic, and political change.

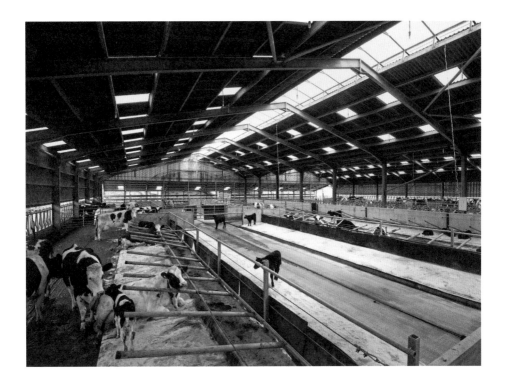

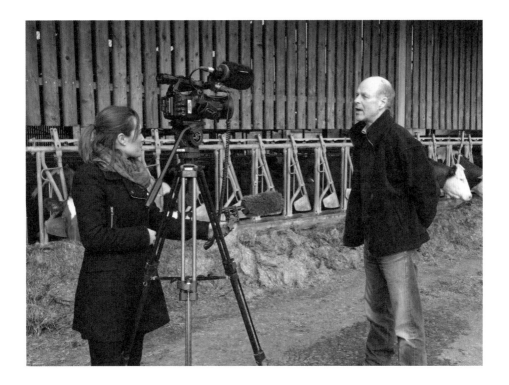

This outlook assumes that farming livestock for food at any level will produce negative outcomes and that the production of food from arable/horticultural sources has little significant environmental, social, or ethical negative impact. However, some studies cast doubt on these assumptions.[4] In fact, the impact of rising global demand for avocados, almonds, and other out-of-season fruit and vegetables is now recognized as having damaging environmental repercussions.

Instinctively, most people would think that farmed ruminant livestock living on naturally grown grass and foraged crops is the best way to produce beef, lamb, and dairy, and I would agree with that. Unfortunately, farmed ruminants have been focused on in the climate change debate as a quick fix. They emit methane, which is twenty-eight times more powerful as a greenhouse gas than carbon,[5] so, it is argued, getting rid of them will cut emissions and buy time to implement other carbon reduction strategies.

However, methane has come from grass-fed ruminants and their rotting grassland vegetation for millennia. It is estimated that the methane from ruminants currently contributes about three per cent to the total greenhouse gas effect and the contribution from grass-fed ruminants (as opposed to those fed grain and soya in intensive systems) has not changed significantly even in recent times.[6] To blame these animals for our current predicament is therefore, in my opinion, wrong and deflects attention from the real culprits – those living in energy intensive, fossil-fuel driven industrial systems. This is where the drive for our farming methods stems from.

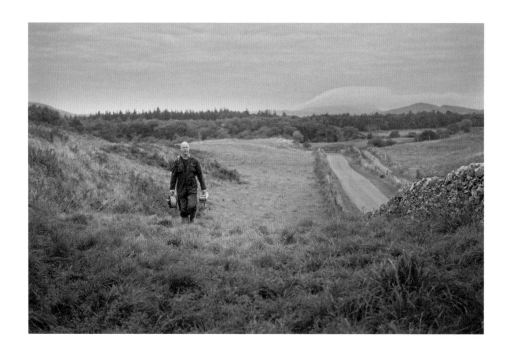

ECOLOGICAL FARMING

I am an ecological farmer, which means I farm in a way that works with nature, not against it. To produce healthy, nutrient-rich food for today and tomorrow, the methods we use on our farm are designed to support human and animal health, while actively improving soil and water quality and increasing biodiversity on the land. This ecological approach to food production throws up the question: 'Can low-impact livestock farming complement arable farming to deliver enough sustainable food?' I think it can.

Ecological models look at ways animals can complement a plant-based food system to utilize co-products,[7] by-products,[8] food waste, and grasslands, while adding fertility to the soils. This is because by utilizing grasslands that are unfit for crop production and arable by-products that humans cannot eat, and by being a fertility-building part of an arable rotation,[9] livestock can add to total global food production. If similar models were adopted globally, meat and dairy production would fall from current levels, but total global food production could then be greater than from crops alone. The release of arable land from the production of animal feed would allow low-impact, plant-based systems to produce the balance of our food requirements for the foreseeable future. These low-impact farming models would be ecologically based and move towards a closed-loop system. Any form of farming involves compromise, but this model can potentially deliver adequate amounts of affordable food while also delivering substantial public benefits and not necessarily at any extra cost to society.

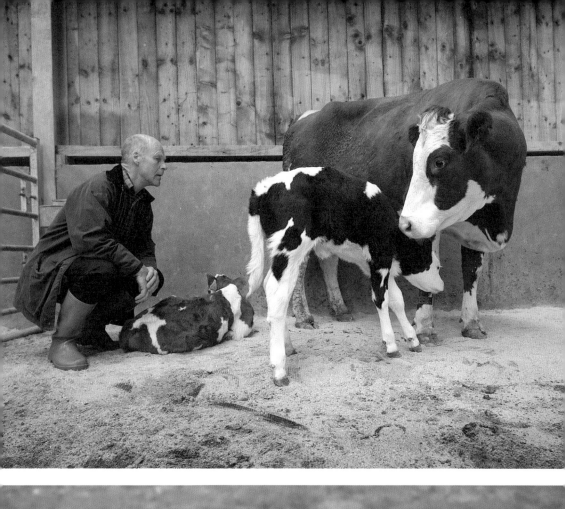

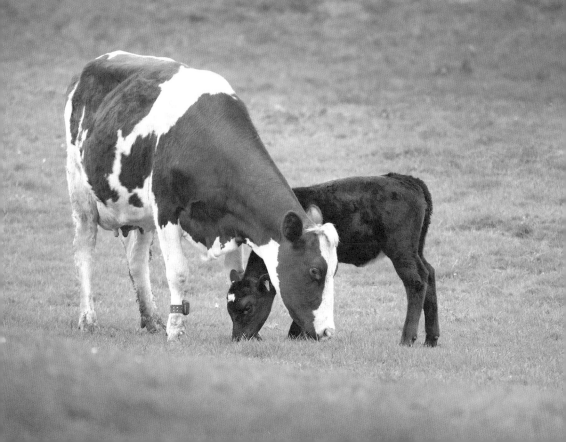

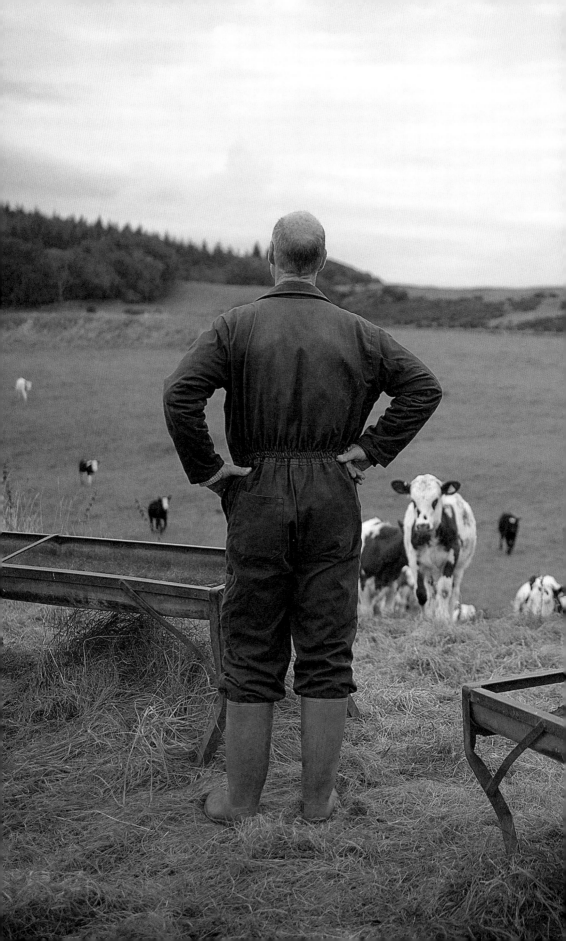

PRIORITIZING BIODIVERSITY

We use the term biodiversity a lot when we talk about our farming system because it is incredibly important to the way we farm here at Rainton. Biodiversity (or biological diversity) is the web of life – the interconnected ecological system that is nature in all its glorious complexity.

There has been a great deal of interest in the media about biodiversity loss – in particular the disappearing insects, butterflies, and birds. There are concerns that biodiversity loss and potential ecological collapse could be a greater threat to humanity than even climate change. We share those concerns. Industrial farming practices, both arable and livestock, have been criticized as a contributing factor to biodiversity loss. Biodiversity on a farm creates an integrated food web where animal, plant, and microbial life largely self-regulate. On monoculture farms – farms that focus on only one crop – biodiversity struggles to exist. Monoculture is typical of large-scale industrial farming.

Increasing biodiversity on our farm has been a priority for us for the last twenty years, as we transitioned to organic farming and planted 35,000 mixed broad-leaved trees on our farm. Our conversion to organic saw the return of farming practices that benefit wildlife rather than threaten it. Every day we can see the difference that prioritizing biodiversity has made. Our planted hedgerows and well-maintained dykes provide a haven for wildlife. We no longer use pesticides or herbicides so wildflowers thrive in our pastures and offer safe refuge to countless bumblebees, dragonflies, and butterflies. Our native woodland provides safe habitat for the endangered red squirrel.

> "Biodiversity (or biological diversity) is the web of life – the interconnected ecological system that is nature in all its glorious complexity"

Our farm is teeming with life and we have worked with environmental organizations to record and document the species that are found on our farm. Following species surveys, two large areas of our farm were designated as Local Wildlife Sites – a nationally recognized designation for areas of land in the UK that are especially important for wildlife.

It is about harnessing the natural system. For example, as mentioned we have an anaerobic digester that turns farm waste into fertilizer and captures methane, which powers a boiler engine that produces electricity and heats water. Housing animals with more space, air, and light reduces their stress and makes them more resilient, which makes them more healthy and productive. Maintaining a balance of clovers means that better grass increases the yield. When we were applying soluble nitrogen to our grasslands and herbicides to kill the perennial weeds, the clovers tended to die out. Clovers are legumes and through a complex method capture nitrogen out of the air and turn it into fertilizer nitrogen that they share with companion plants. All of these little things work together.

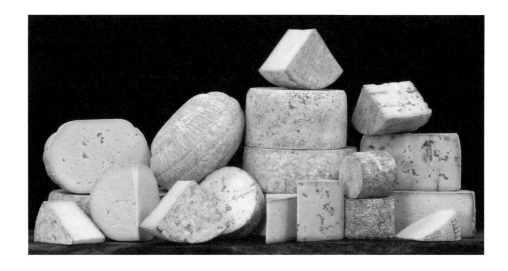

EMBRACING A NEW SCIENCE

It saddens me to hear people lambasting organic farming as being 'anti-science' when I now farm in a fashion that requires a far deeper understanding of the parasites and diseases and the effects of management systems on animal behaviour (and in turn on production performance) than I ever did when I blindly followed the prescriptive protocols of intensive farming. Looking back and comparing our system now with how we farmed in our more intensive period (and even that wasn't particularly intensive by many standards) confirms my belief that the certainty of our industry's intensification mantra has been thoroughly undermined.

Most farmers are caught between a rock and a hard place between the expensive supply industry (machinery, fertilizers, agrochemicals, and antibiotics) and the retailers who want to make profit. Government policy tends to be cheap food and exports. This often means that individual farmers are overworked farming 1,000 dairy cows housed for a 365-day winter. It is causing burnout in farmers and in animals, and the land is covered in slurry because you have to get rid of it somehow.

Since the early 2000s, we at Rainton Farm have created new ponds and broad-leaved woodlands on ten per cent of the farm while increasing the productivity of the remaining ninety per cent through, for example, red clovers, reseeding, and use of digestate. Our farm production in recent years has matched that of the 1990s, when we applied all those agrochemicals to our land and our animals. It is estimated that we have improved our farm biodiversity by around 400 per cent overall while at the same time our total farm agricultural output has increased by over ten per cent. How far can we and the rest of the farming world take this ecological model? We have seen our farm profitability grow due mainly to the enormous cost saving. We are still exploring what is possible, but with each day that passes we see the clear benefits of this approach – over a ninety per cent reduction of soluble fertilizers, pesticides, vaccines, and antibiotics, a fifty per cent reduction in carbon emissions, doubling the working life of our cows, reducing the working hours of our staff, increasing net food production, and maintaining a profitable business.

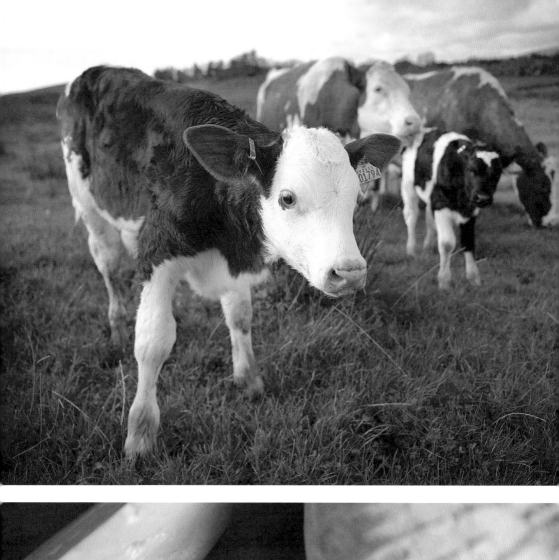

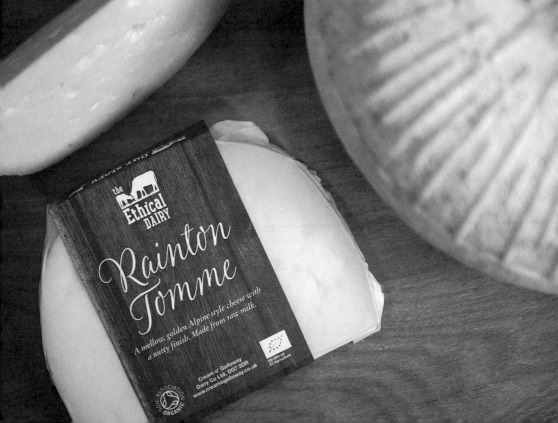

the
Ethical DAIRY

Rainton Tomme

A mellow, golden Alpine-style cheese with
a nutty finish. Made from raw milk.

Cream o' Galloway
Dairy Co Ltd. DG7 2DR
www.creamogalloway.co.uk

GB-ORG-05
EU Agriculture

SOIL ASSOCIATION ORGANIC

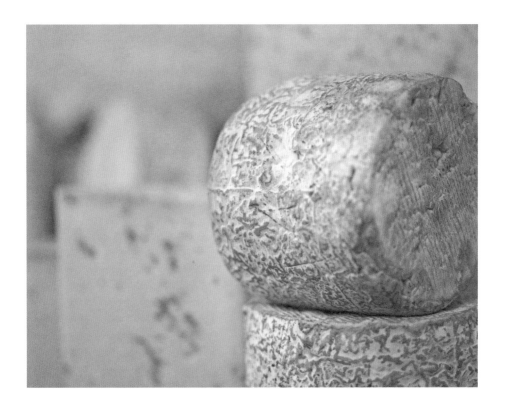

THE BENEFITS OF RAW-MILK CHEESE

Our cheese is raw-milk cheese, meaning it is made from milk that has not been pasteurized. Unpasteurized cheese has long been recognized as having greater depth and complexity of flavour than pasteurized cheese, and it is increasingly becoming valued as a natural source of probiotics. Science is now showing that raw-milk cheese has a complex microbial biome that is heavily influenced by the bacteria in the cow's milk, which, in turn, is influenced by the bacteria on the cow, which relates to the bacteria in the food the cow eats, which is greatly influenced by the microbes in the soil the crops have been grown on. If the whey from that cheese is fed to pigs and their muck is returned to the soil, all on the same farm, we have a closed-loop bacterial cycle, producing a cheese that is unique to that farm. That is the concept behind the old description of a cheese's 'terroir'.

Healthy soils, crops, and cows substantially reduce the risk of pathogens and also the need for sterilization. There is now growing evidence that our over-processed, sterile food system is creating imbalances in our bodies' microbe community and in turn in our immune systems, resulting in associated long-term well-being and health issues. This is why there is growing interest in the health benefits from consuming naturally fermented foods – raw-milk cheese being among these. And it is why we have opted to make raw-milk cheeses.

"The ultimate aim is to make a cheese with a healthy balance of microorganisms"

However, we have faced resistance from food and public health establishments over safety concerns. There will always be a risk, but with the help of modern science and technology, that risk can be managed. We test extensively for pathogen presence, yet the need for wholesale food sterilization is, I believe, unnecessary and is potentially contributing to the recent rises in long-term food-related illnesses. We don't need to damage good, wholesome food that is actively stimulating our inner biome and consequently our health and our well-being.

There is a lot of collaborative work among farmers and cheesemakers worldwide to help advance the understanding of how we can increase the diversity of good bacteria in cheese. Instead of thinking that unpasteurized cheese is taking a step backwards, where food safety might be compromised, farmers and cheesemakers are working together to understand how we can improve the bacteria in the soil, which then transfer to the grass to the cows and the milk. The ultimate aim is to make a cheese with a healthy balance of microorganisms.

HOW IS CHEESE MADE?

We make cheese in a very traditional way. We begin with milk straight from the cow then add a culture of bacteria to the warm milk, which curdles the milk. The next step is to add rennet – we always use a vegetarian rennet – which turns the milk culture into a jelly-like consistency. Once it has set, the cheese is cut into cubes; generally speaking, the smaller the cubes, the harder the cheese. We let it settle and the whey liquid separates from the curd. Then we drain off the whey, leaving the curds in the vat. For some of our cheeses we add salt at this stage.

Depending on which cheese we are making, we will either put the curds into moulds straight away, or we will 'cheddar' them – a process that brings the loose curds together into blocks and then puts the blocks through a mill to break them back up into smaller pieces. These pieces are then put into the moulds. Some of our cheeses are put on a cheese press to apply weight that firms up the cheese; other types of cheese simply drain under their own weight and are turned regularly during the first few days to ensure an even consistency.

One of the most underappreciated parts of cheese-making is the ageing process. All cheeses need regular turning to maintain an even distribution (and avoid an 'elephant's foot' shaped cheese). Cheese needs a constant temperature, between 8 and 14 °C, and high humidity. Our cave-like stores provide just that.

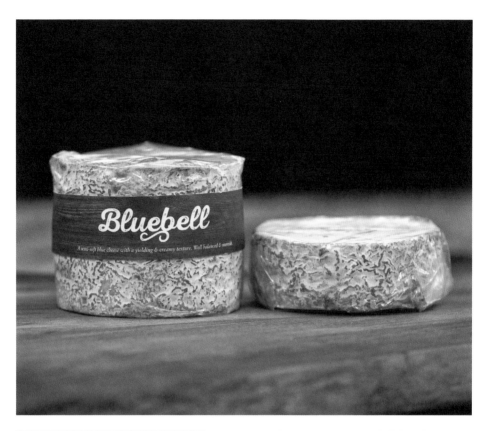

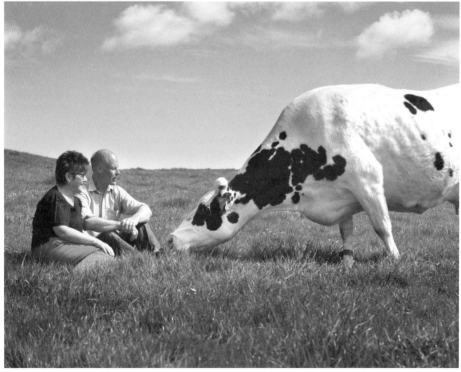

UPSCALING OUR BUSINESS

We have been taken aback at the demand for our cheese since we launched The Ethical Dairy in 2018. Members of the public are crying out for alternatives to intensive food production and our industry needs to respond to that demand. We have used social media to connect with this audience. We did not change our farming system simply due to customer demand – we have been working towards this cow-with-calf farming system for many years. However, the launch of The Ethical Dairy seems to have coincided with growing unease about the dairy industry from members of the public. For many people with concerns about conventional dairy farming, our approach is meeting a need.

During much of 2018 we were running short of cheese as demand for our product exhausted our ability to supply it. Over the winter of 2018/2019 we renovated an old, disused building on the farm to create a larger cheese production space and cheese store. This allows the cheese to be produced in larger batch sizes, which will mean it will be more economically sustainable, and it will mean we have a much larger space to mature the cheese.

> "We are driven by the belief that by rethinking the farming industry, we can produce nutritious food and comfortably feed our population without destroying the environment"

We had always planned to scale up, but the demand from the public meant we needed to do that earlier than intended. To help make this happen, we launched a crowdfunding campaign in autumn 2018, which was successful in raising the money we needed to speed up our expansion plans. At the time of writing, we are putting the finishing touches to the new cheese dairy and will soon be able to make enough cheese to meet existing customer demand. Our long-term goal is to use all the milk produced on the farm for cheese and ice cream production, moving away from reliance on wholesale milk markets completely.

It is very difficult, and extremely expensive, to transition an existing commercial-sized dairy farm to our model of cow-with-calf dairy farming. Other farmers are watching what we do with interest and, while I am sure there are some who are hoping we fail, others are seeing a possible escape from the intensification race. We are supporting a few farmers to pilot the system by providing hands-on training and technical support to them and also to research institutes throughout Europe. In 2019 we organized and hosted the first-ever Ethical Farming Conference, which brought together 200 farmers, researchers, academics, and students from Finland, Sweden, the Netherlands, Ireland, the USA, and the UK, all dedicated to the emerging 'ethical' farming sector. This was an incredible event and we hope it will be the first of many conventions to help catalyse a move towards more morally conscious farming.

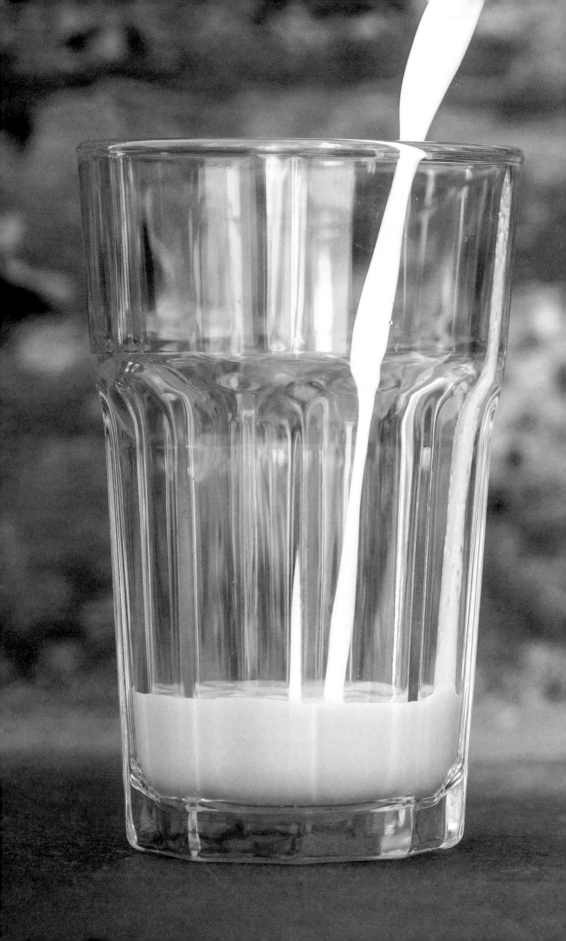

KEFIR

Kefir is a probiotic drink made from milk and is known to offer a plethora of health benefits, particularly those relating to digestion. It is inherently a heritage product by its very nature, passed down from family to family for thousands of years. In the Black Caucasus Mountains where it originated, the tribal villagers jealously guarded their grains, refusing to share them with outsiders. Finally, the Russian government had to send an armed party into the mountains to obtain some of the grains! Kefir is now a billion-euro industry in Russia and Eastern Europe and has spread all over the world. Because wild kefir is a synergistic natural combination of multiple strains of bacteria and yeast, it is far more powerful than any human-made probiotic, which only contains a few strains of bacteria.

"We first became enchanted with kefir when we began to understand that the microbiome inside us is just the same as the ecosystem outside us – filled with beautiful, biodiverse life forms that need to be cherished and nourished"

Shann Jones, Chuckling Goat

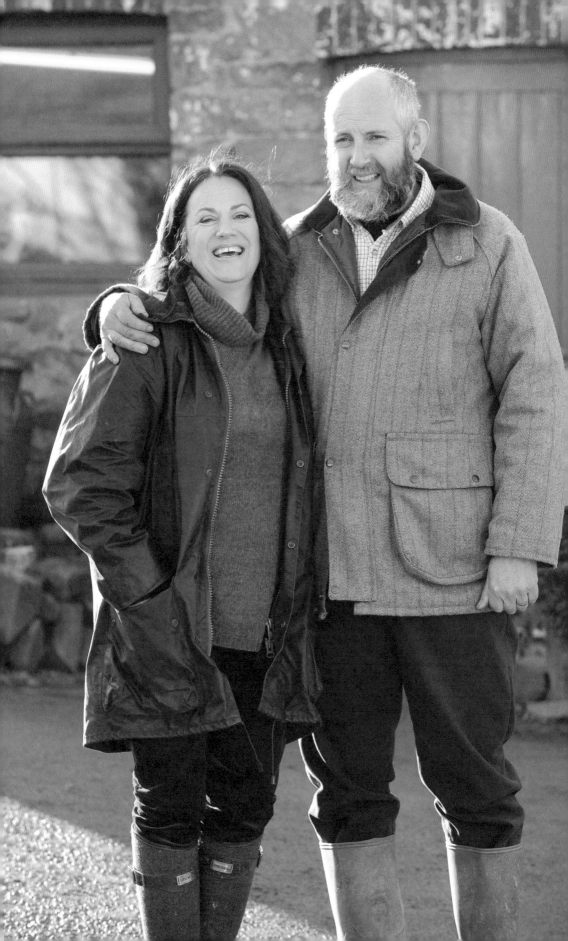

CHUCKLING GOAT

SHANN & RICHARD JONES

South West Wales, UK | chucklinggoat.co.uk

Our story is a true necessity-is-the-mother-of-invention tale. As a former radio talk show host and a former harp maker, we were driven to innovate with natural answers when our family had health issues and conventional medicine was not achieving the results we wanted. We bought our first goat because our little boy Benji suffered from eczema and bronchial problems. Course after course of antibiotics was creating a vicious spiral, leaving him sicker each time. Ancient Welsh knowledge holds that goats' milk is helpful for these issues, and Rich, as a Welsh farmer, understood that. So, we began milking the goat, and although the milk helped Benji's bronchial condition, we soon had too much leftover goats' milk. In order to use up the surplus, Shann learned how to make a Russian probiotic drink called kefir.

Then, in 2012, Rich contracted a life-threatening MRSA infection. With no other recourse, we used the kefir to help clear his infection. This experience taught us that kefir works as effectively on the skin as it does inside the gut, and we began to experiment with adding the kefir to soaps and lotions. Today, Chuckling Goat has pioneered a protocol that combines drinking kefir with kefir skincare to achieve results on eczema, psoriasis, rosacea, and acne, as well as IBS, depression, anxiety, and allergies. Our kefir is also included in the College of Obstetricians 'Mum Plus One' initiative, which will be rolled out to 600,000 pregnant women beginning 2020.

A MICROBIOME

Everything that we sell in the business today started out in our farmhouse kitchen. We fermented our initial batch of kefir in a Kilner jar on the kitchen windowsill. We first became enchanted with kefir when we began to understand that the microbiome inside us is just the same as the ecosystem outside of us – filled with beautiful, biodiverse life forms that need to be cherished and nourished.

We learned this lesson on the farm, watching our compost heap. We would feed the goats our own hay, milk them, and muck out their stalls. The muck went onto the compost heap, and was broken down into rich, crumbly, natural DOM (dissolved organic matter) fertilizer by the ministrations of trillions of tiny magical creatures. The DOM fertilizer went back onto our ancient, deep-rooted wildflower hay fields to enrich the hay, which we mow, bale, and feed to the goats. This rotating wheel of production secures us into a graceful cycle of sustainability – power supplied by micro-agents in the muck. It became apparent that our inner-gut ecosystems are exactly the same as the ones in the muck heap! The job of microorganisms in both instances is breaking down the raw ingredients they are given into a usable energy source.

> "Bringing the whole system into balance, by using live helpful bacteria, is the answer, both for the microbiomes inside us, and the macrobiomes on the planet around us"

Relating to your own gut, or to the planet around you, is the same action, and requires the same rules of engagement: Love it. Feed it. Don't poison it. Kefir grains are living organisms and feeding them milk is the same process as looking after our goats on the farm. We feed the goats – and the kefir grains – and look after them, and they give us their wonderful, life-serving bounty. I imagine the kefir grains like tiny herd animals; keeping kefir on the windowsill is like having a little farm in a jar.

The real breakthrough for us came when we began to understand that your skin is also a biome – a wild jungle of life forms – that also needs to be fed and cherished. Antibacterial soaps, for example, kill off good bacteria in the skin biome the same way that antibiotics kill off good bugs in the gut biome. Like pouring bleach into the river, these toxic substances kill everything – not just the bad guys that you are trying to attack. Good health is in part about filling the space with the right things – you need to proactively put those good bugs into the system, in both gut and skin biomes, rather than emptying the space with antibiotics and antibacterial cleaners, which allow the bad bacteria to jump into the void that you have created. I believe that killing the bad bugs is not the way forward. Bringing the whole system into balance, by using live helpful bacteria, is the answer, both for the microbiomes inside us, and the macrobiomes on the planet around us.

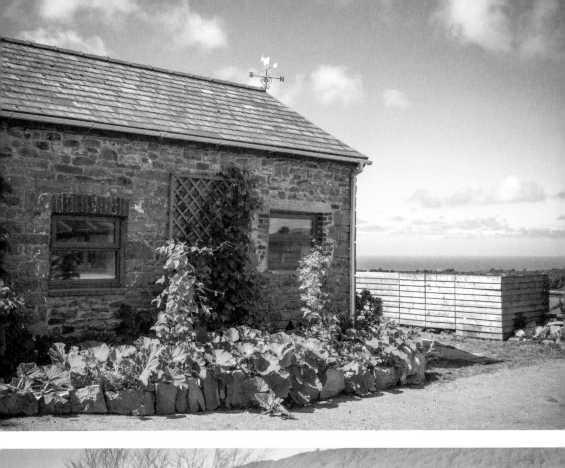
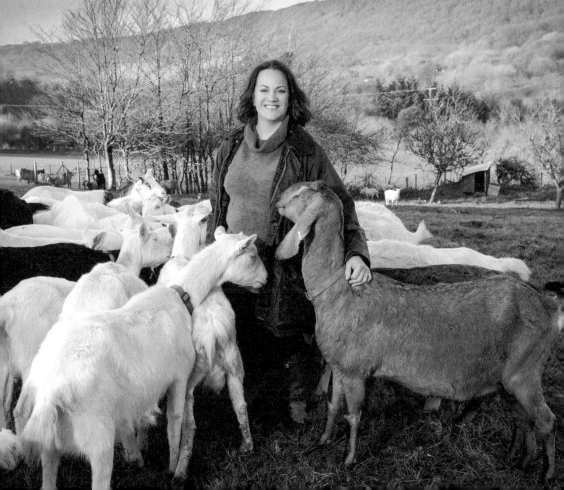

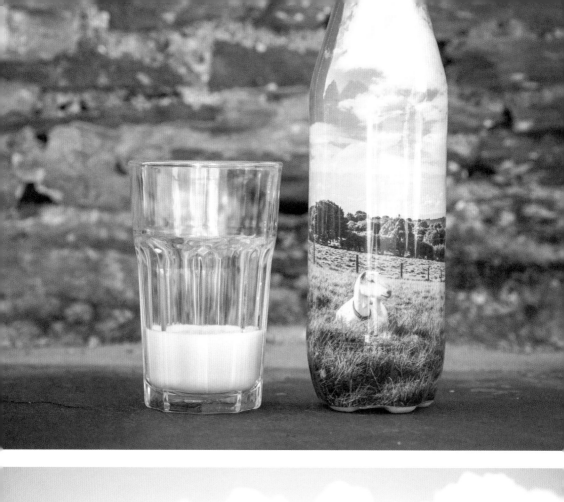

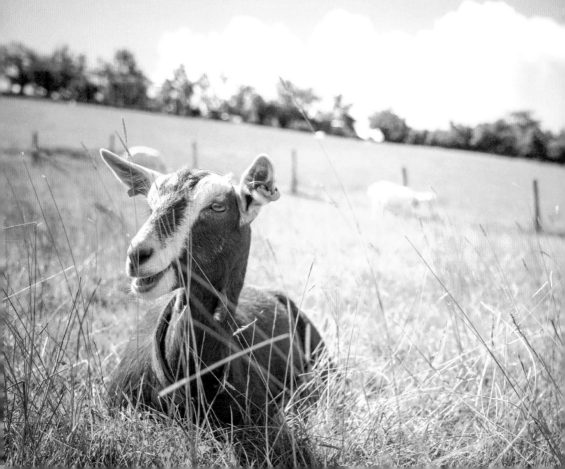

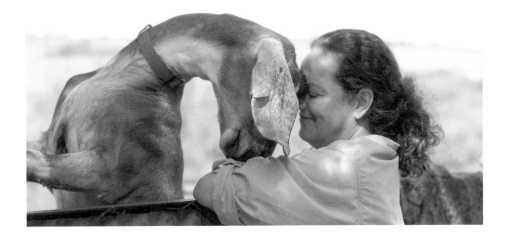

A JOURNEY OF EDUCATION

Kefir tells an amazing story – from its mysterious origin in the Black Caucasus Mountains to its gradual spread across the globe. When I began this journey, almost no one in the UK had heard of kefir. I heard about it from a Russian doctor, who was discussing it on the radio. I realized very early on that my mission was going to be one of education, rather than trying to sell a product. I became a bit like Dr Seuss' *Horton Hears a Who* – an ever-so-slightly eccentric advocate for an entire tiny world that no one could see, and very few people besides myself seemed to care about.

Most people said: 'I have bugs inside me? Bugs – ick!' 'NOT ick!' I insisted. 'Bugs – yay!' Bugs are beautiful. Love your gut bugs! Think of them as a magnificent Amazon rainforest – birds, fish, flowers, trees, leaves, deer, jaguar. There is an entire world in there, all dependent on you for their food source. Cooperate with them – or everyone suffers.

In the beginning, no one knew what I was talking about, and I got some very strange looks. But as I continued to press forward, the message started to penetrate. I began to hear other people mentioning the Amazon rainforest metaphor, and asking questions about kefir and what it could do for them. That is when our business really began to take off.

At the same time as building an awareness of the benefits of kefir, it is important to us that we are in direct communication with our customers, because drinking kefir is not always a straightforward process. It is very strong and can create a negative detox effect if clients increase the amount too quickly. Information and contact are as important as the kefir itself – we are looking to educate people to become good stewards of their own gut microbiomes, so maintaining a close relationship with them is critical.

THE ALCHEMY OF KEFIR

We ensure that everything is sustainably sourced by keeping our processes very simple. The only things needed for the kefir are goats' milk – which we source from a Red Tractor assured farm[10] – and our own kefir grains, which we grow and tend in-house. We buy our bottles from a UK distributor, and keep everything as close to home as we possibly can. All our packaging is recyclable, and we use compostable starch chips to fill our boxes.

01 Sourcing the milk The best milk for kefir is goats' milk, as cows' milk contains the inflammatory A1 casein, which can be allergenic. In the beginning, we milked our own goats. As our business grew, we partnered with St Helen's Farm in Yorkshire to bring in milk to supplement our own, as our own goats couldn't keep up with demand.

02 Kefir grains Real kefir is made with kefir grains, which are living organisms that are a constellation of multiple strains of beneficial yeasts and bacteria. Different kefir grains have different bio-profiles, which are affected by what they are fed and how they are kept.

03 Fermentation The kefir grains do all the work here; they are essentially 'eating' the milk, working their way through the natural fats, sugars, and proteins, converting the milk into something similar to a drinking yogurt. You will come across more of these kinds of micro-processes occurring throughout this book, for example those that occur in soil, which Charles Dowding talks about on p. 180 – there are many great examples of nature breaking things down to create something beneficial to other organisms.

04 Stirring The kefir needs to be stirred at least three times a day; this breaks the crust on top and allows kefir grains to access fresh milk. Because kefir is acidic, it is important to use silicone or stainless-steel implements only – no aluminium or inferior metals.

05 Testing the pH level Kefir is a natural fermented food; the way that you know it is safe and ready to drink is when the pH drops to 3.7 or below. It is important that the pH is reduced to 4.5 or lower within the first eighteen hours of fermentation – any slower than this, and you run the risk of spoilage bacteria entering the milk. We check the pH of our kefir once at eighteen hours and again at thirty-six hours. The speed of the fermentation is controlled by the ambient temperature of the room (heat speeds up the process) as well as the ratio of grains to milk (the more grains in the mix, the faster the fermentation).

SHARING THE HEALTH

Kefir grains grow and replicate over time, so if you look after them properly, they will live as long as you do, and you should never need to repurchase. You can even give the extra grains away to friends! In Ireland there is a tradition that kefir grains are the 'health' of the family, and when a son gets married, his mother gives a handful of grains to the new wife.

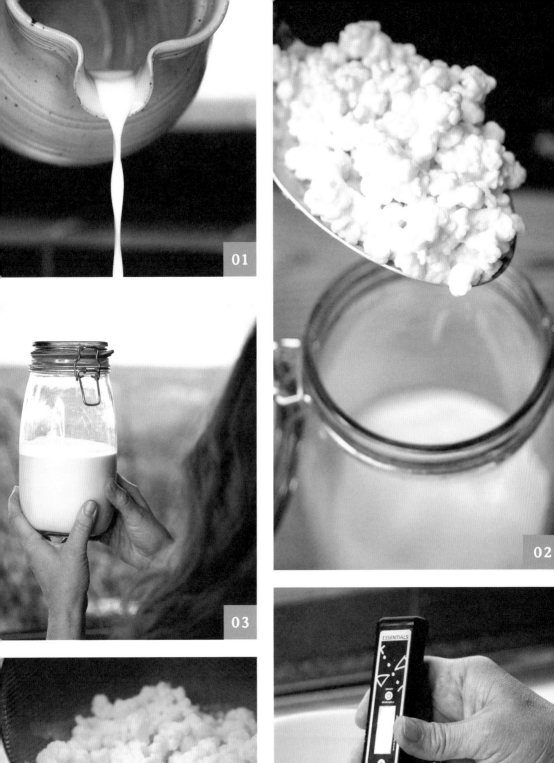

01

02

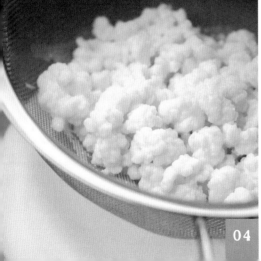

03

04

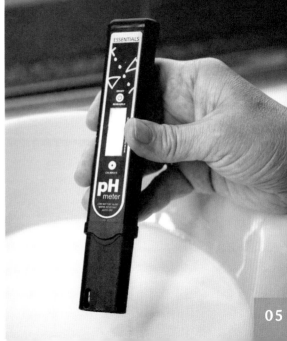

05

06 Straining The kefir grains are then strained and set aside as they are not consumed – they are starter organisms only, which is why they can be passed on and reused, like in a sourdough bread process.

07 Regularly testing the microbiology Reusing live cultures can be a fantastic boon for human health, but can also bring attendant risk. Kefir grains are living organisms, and just like humans, they can contract viruses. This is called 'bacteriaphage' (or phage, for short). If phage contaminates kefir grains and those grains are continually reused, the contamination can spread and grow, resulting in potentially lethal food poisoning. At Chuckling Goat we have our kefir regularly testing by a food safety lab. If you are making kefir at home, we strongly recommend you do the same.

08 Packaging These days, we bottle and cap our kefir in the dairy. In the beginning we used a pouring jug, but we now have a bottling machine and a capping machine. However, this process is not highly automated – we prefer to hire local people, and pay them well, rather than purchase an expensive machine. South West Wales is an economically challenged area, so creating good local jobs matters to us.

THE QUESTION OF PLASTIC

You will notice that we use plastic bottles rather than glass. We have looked carefully into the packaging issue. We found that shipping glass ultimately has five times the total carbon footprint when compared to shipping recyclable plastic because of the additional weight and production burden. It is therefore not a viable option for our system. The kefir is very active, so needs to be contained in strong packaging. The moment that technology produces a better option than plastic for our process, we will jump on it!

09 Boxing and shipping We box the products and ship directly to our customers. We do not sell through any distributors; we only send direct to the end user. In today's business environment, I believe that the golden standard is communication with the customer. Whatever business you are in, you are in the relationship business. It is this relationship with the customer that matters to me.

We never wanted to just sell a product – our intention was always to create natural health solutions for people who wanted to improve their health. However, natural healing is a slow process, and not always straightforward, so as mentioned on p. 71 it is important that we are in direct contact with our customers, so that we can coach them through the process.

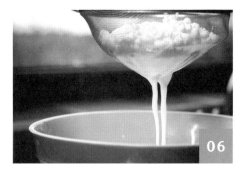
06

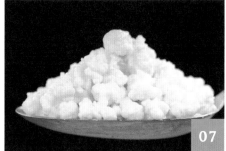
07

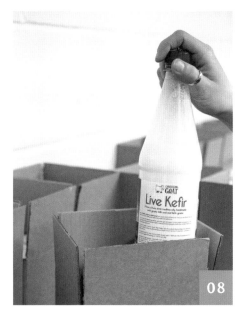
08

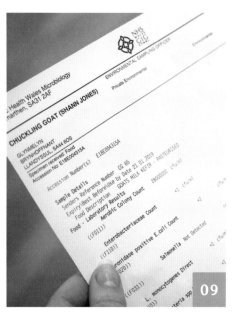
09

MEETING FOOD HYGIENE STANDARDS

One of our challenges is that kefir is a relatively novel food in the UK, and so we have been working closely with Environmental Health to help it develop the proper scientific protocols for testing. Our hygiene requirements are stringent – we have a perfect level 5 hygiene rating, and we work hard to keep it that way. When we started, we were making kefir in a stone barn, and we had to be creative to find ways to keep it spotless without losing the character of the old farm building. These days we make the kefir in our shiny new workshop, which Rich custom-designed for the purpose. It is a lot easier to keep clean than the old outbuildings.

Any time you work with food, your processes have to be impeccable. We are regularly inspected by Environmental Health, and our paperwork load is intense. We do computerized swab testing, and regularly send our kefir off for microbiological testing. We use a lot of modern technology and cutting-edge science to make sure that our traditional product is up to modern hygiene standards.

A FAMILY-RUN BUSINESS

Today, our tiny kitchen-table business has grown beyond recognition. We started out with just Rich and me; now we have twenty-two employees, hundreds of thousands of customers, and we ship all over the world. In 2014, Rich had to sell his motorcycle to raise the funds for us to buy bottles to put the kefir in. Now we are a multi-million-pound enterprise, with a growth rate of 6,000% between 2014 and 2019. Sometimes it is exciting – and sometimes it is just crazy! Alongside our drinking kefir we also sell a range of kefir-based skincare products.

These days our daughter, Elen, runs the office, and her husband, Josh, is our production manager. Rich's brother, Rhys, is our groundskeeper. We love working with our family close around us. Developing the business to the point where we can afford to provide employment for so many family members is one of our proudest achievements. With our skincare products, we are a complete end-to-end business – we grow the hay, mow the hay, feed the goats, milk the goats, and create the products. With the milk we get from St Helen's, we make the kefir, bottle it up, box it, ship it out, and handle customer issues. We have now invested in a labelling machine, so we can label our bottles ourselves as well. We have found that no one cares as much as we do about making our products immaculate. For that reason, the more processes we can do in-house, the better things go.

Today, we have personally trained a team of top communicators in the farm's office, and we manage our entire global customer base from there, using phone, email, and the live chat function on our website. Shann is in our open-plan office four days a week, ready to jump on the phone as needed, and has shifted her attention to innovating new products, writing books (such as *The Essential Book of Gut Health for Mum, Bump and Baby*, published by Hay House, 2020), and consulting with clients who have particularly tricky health issues. Meanwhile, Rich manages the farm and does ongoing maintenance and development of the physical buildings and equipment.

> "If you create a beautiful, high-quality product, and stay true to your values, customers will seek you out"

We are busy all year round, but we do have slower periods – December, for example, is a slow month for us because our product is therapeutic, and no one wants to think about gut health while they are trying to enjoy themselves during the festive season. But we make up for it in January, when everyone is trying to clean up and get healthy again after their festive excesses.

To anyone who is starting out, I would say: stick with your passion. Never compromise. Never cut corners. Keep it immaculate. The world is already too full of mass-produced, low-quality food. If you create a beautiful, high-quality product, and stay true to your values, customers will seek you out.

CULTIVATING AN ENVIRONMENT OF CARE

We start the day with a full team meeting at 8.00 am. We sit in a circle, and everyone shares something about how they're feeling, and what's going on in their lives. As a small, tightly knit team, we work together so closely that I think it is critical that everyone knows how everyone else is feeling. These daily meetings contribute to our team alignment and high performance.

We finish the day at 4.00 pm, so people can go home and be with their families. Our company motto is 'Family first'. No one has ever laid on their deathbed wishing they had spent more time at work! This outlook has given us a team of workers who are passionate about our company and what we do. Last Christmas every member of the team got a £1,000 bonus. I can't think of anything more important to do with our profits than make our team feel valued for all their hard work.

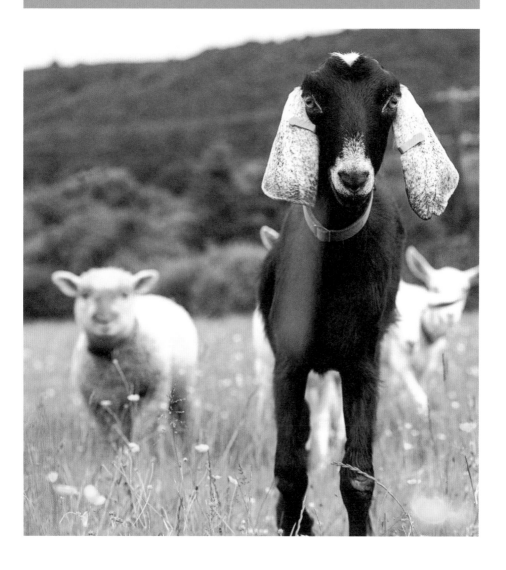

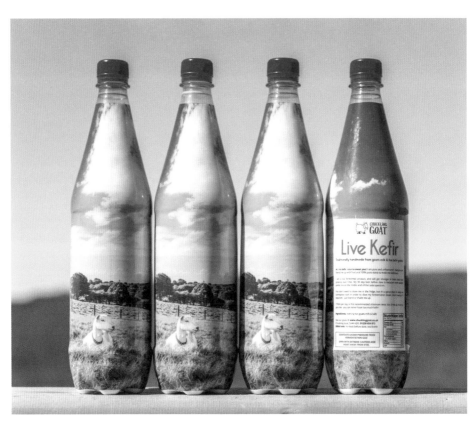

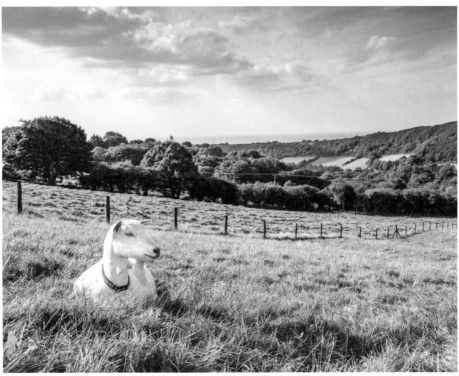

BALANCING TRADITION
AND MODERNITY

We did have a shop in the local town of Cardigan for a while but decided to close it down. Most of our business is now online. We don't have a shop as such now, although we do help people who turn up at the farm wanting to know more about our products. We pour all available resources into our website, which is as powerful, fast, and beautiful as we can possibly make it. We make up for the lack of physical access by offering free shipping across the UK. Personally, I believe that bricks and mortar is dead. The fact that you can order nearly anything in the entire world, and have it appear on your doorstep the next day, has changed everything, forever. We have tried to marry this technology to our small-scale, handmade approach, and we have had great success. I believe new technology can be a great boon to small producers, if they embrace it. Online is the perfect place for a niche product.

Social media has also been very important for us. Back in the days when we were broke, we exclusively used social media because we had no budget for anything else. Now that we can afford some advertising budget, we still value social media as a powerful way to communicate with our customers and answer questions.

> "Like the power of nature itself, kefir is more than the sum of its parts. I feel truly privileged to work with this amazing, health-promoting substance"

However, it is vital to us that we are both high-tech and high-touch. Despite the fact that we are focused on our website, we are very determined to keep everything human scale. Instead of having a huge vat where we process the kefir, we use multiple small microbrewery vats, which can be lifted and cleaned by one person. Instead of having a lot of automation on site, we use our resources to create a lot of high-quality local jobs. Our starting rate for an entry level position is substantially higher than minimum wage, and we offer regular salary raises and promotions.

Traditionally made kefir is a special thing; most companies use a powdered kefir starter, instead of live kefir grains. For this reason, competition from supermarkets is not really an issue for us, because large commercial outlets don't offer what we offer. Using real grains brings its own challenges, however – they can be tricky and demanding. Looking after them is more like farming than manufacturing, because they are living organisms. But we have a relationship with our grains, just as we do all the bigger animals on the farm, so that makes it worthwhile for us. Using live grains creates a powerful, active product that should not be pasteurized before it reaches the final user. Like the power of nature itself, kefir is more than the sum of its parts. I feel truly privileged to work with this amazing, health-promoting substance.

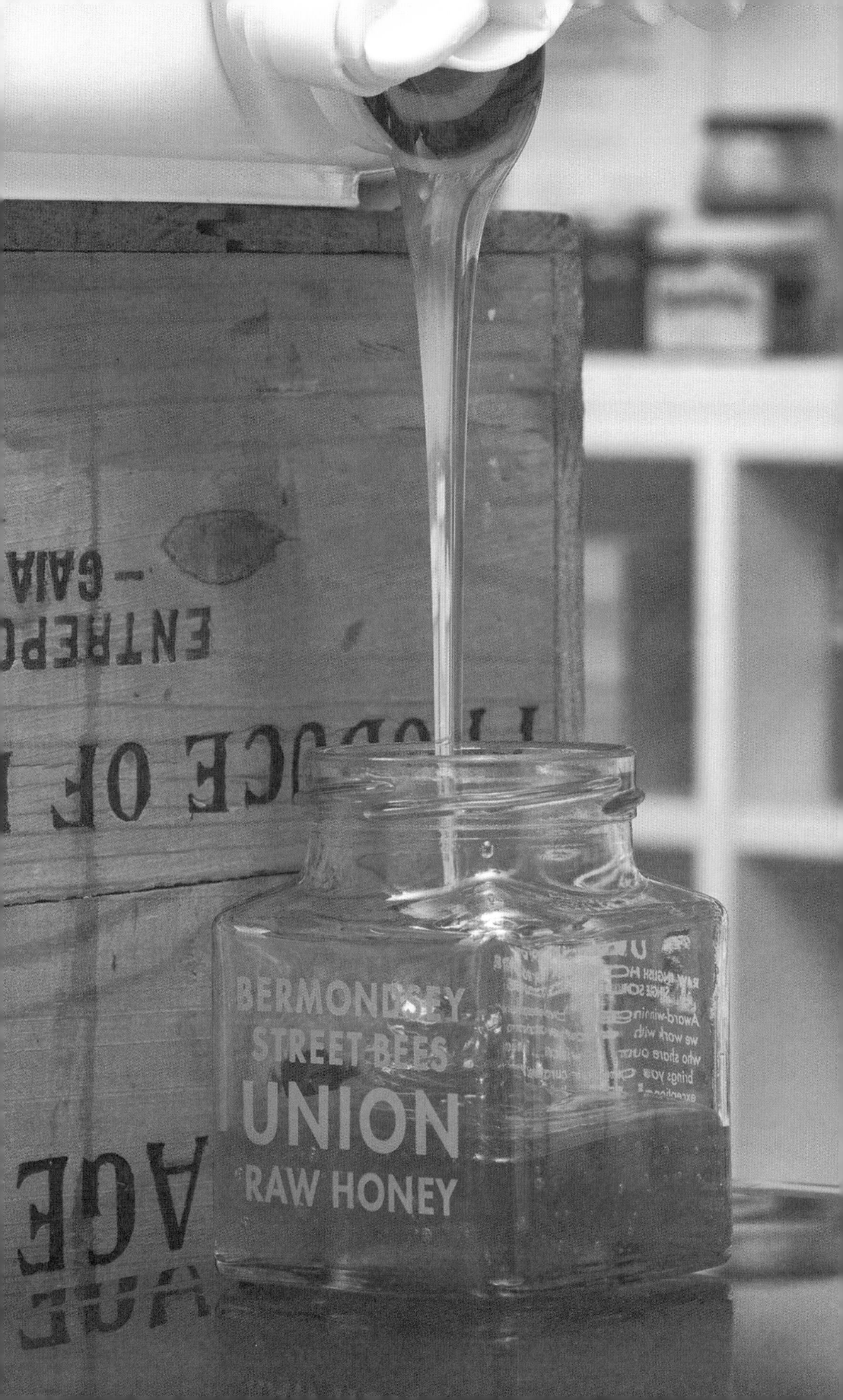
BERMONDSEY
STREET BEES
UNION
RAW HONEY

HONEY

Honey is a natural and nutritious food that has been made by honeybees for millions of years. It can vary wildly in flavour depending on the nectar of the flowers it was made from. Acting as an excellent sugar substitute and a versatile component of many sweet and savoury recipes, in both its natural and raw form, honey is thought to have numerous health benefits due to its antibacterial and antioxidant properties.

"Beekeeping and the production of raw honey is an ancient craft; we feel our connection with this tradition very powerfully"

Dale Gibson & Sarah Wyndham Lewis, Bermondsey Street Bees

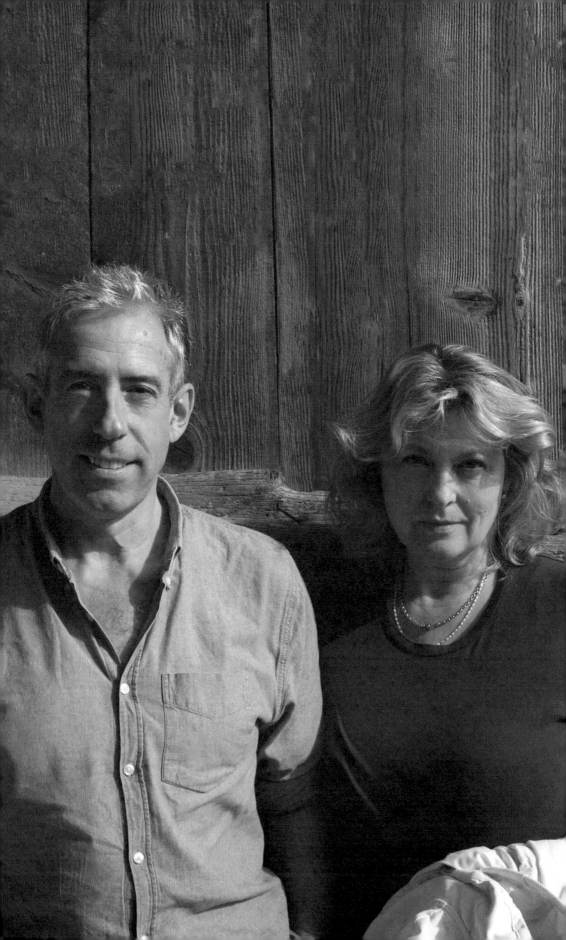

BERMONDSEY STREET BEES

DALE GIBSON & SARAH WYNDHAM LEWIS

London, UK | bermondseystreetbees.co.uk

Bermondsey Street Bees was founded in 2007. Two years earlier, we had moved into a Victorian warehouse just around the corner from London's historic Borough Market. One of our first missions while finding our feet there was to find an allotment. It was there that some honeybees caught Dale's attention one day. He came home desperate to know more about them and a couple of weeks later we found ourselves among the great and good of London's beekeepers at an introduction day. This was the beginning of everything: Dale began his training shortly afterwards under the mentorship of the famous John Chapple, the Queen's beekeeper. With some solid experience under Dale's belt, we became proud caretakers of first one rooftop hive and then a second. At that stage, Dale was still a stockbroker working in the City, but the bees had other plans. Gradually, the number of hive sites expanded as he became more and more experienced. His reputation as a highly principled beekeeper grew and we won several significant prizes, including 'Best Honey in London' in 2011.

Two extraordinary events finally tipped the balance, transforming Bermondsey Street Bees from busy hobbyist beekeepers into a full-time business. In 2014, Michelin-starred chef Tom Aikens asked us to establish bees for him in the kitchen garden of the new Soho Farmhouse in Oxfordshire as part of a carefully constructed ecosystem. And in 2016, we were awarded 'UK Small Artisan Producer of The Year' at the Great Taste Awards – the food equivalent of winning an Oscar. For us, the most exciting part of the award was that it recognized both our skill as honey producers and the significance of the sustainability agenda we had set since our very earliest days as beekeepers.

THE ART OF BEEKEEPING

There are so many different ways of approaching beekeeping. For some people, it is all about honey as a commodity crop or the potential to be paid for intensive pollination services. In this mechanistic scenario, the bees simply serve as mankind's lowly servants. At the other end of the scale, you have passionate 'natural beekeepers' propounding an entirely hands-off approach in a noble effort to pay bees the greatest possible respect. Neither of these extremes represents our best chance of maintaining managed or wild bee populations in the modern world.

Complicating everything further still, there is an enormous amount of misinformation in the popular understanding of bees. For a start, what actually *is* a honeybee? There are more than 20,000 species of bee in the world – of which only *seven* are honeybees, uniquely defined by the fact that they store food (honey) in their nest (hive) to allow them to overwinter or survive tough times as an intact colony.

Environmental changes and pressures mean that there are almost no wild honeybees left in the developed world. This puts the weight of maintaining stocks of these essential pollinators firmly on the shoulders of beekeepers, whether hobbyists or commercial set-ups. And, as with anything else in the world, there are good and bad practitioners in both sectors.

For us, the greatest joy in what we do is the platform it gives us to educate and to develop templates for responsible, sustainable beekeeping. Beekeeping and the production of raw honey is an ancient craft; we feel our connection with this tradition very powerfully, but we also know that in the modern world good beekeepers have to be savvy scientists. Only if we analyse and understand what is afflicting our bees – and share this knowledge – do we have any future. So, education is a key element of our work and takes us all over the world, sharing knowledge with a fascinating variety of people.

WHAT IS HONEY?

Honeybees produce honey as stores to allow them to overwinter as a colony. This behaviour is unique to the honeybee. The base component of honey is the nectar that the honeybees bring into the colony from flowers, which can be as much as seventy per cent water. The bees process the nectar through their bodies, changing the nature of the sugars. Finally, the nectar is evaporated down to around eighteen per cent water through the fanning of the bees' wings and stored in the comb as honey. Each hexagonal cell is then capped with wax to preserve it indefinitely, until the bees need to access it to feed the colony through winter or other hard times.

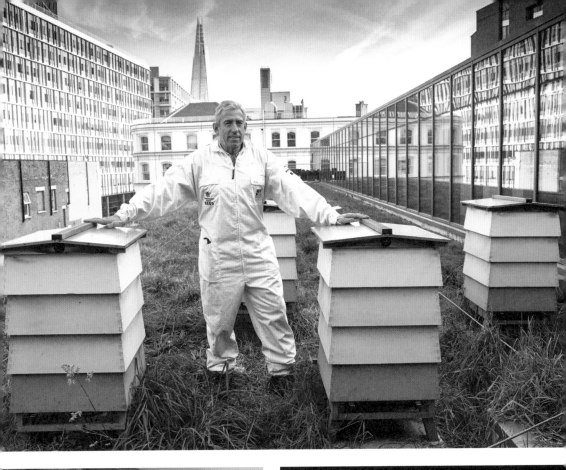

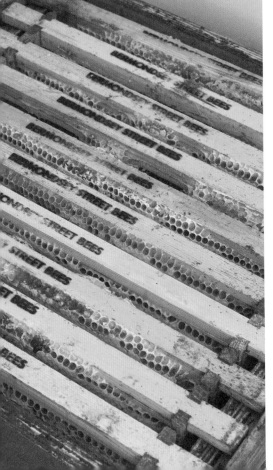

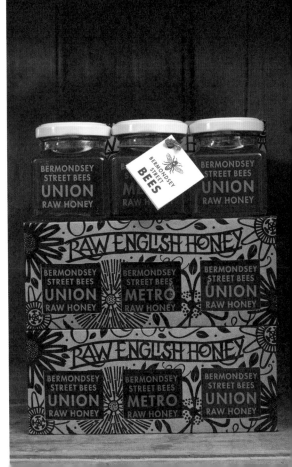

HEALTHY BEES, HEALTHY HONEY

Worldwide research into the causes of declining honeybee numbers always throws up the same fundamental conclusion – that the lack of natural habitat/forage is what crucially undermines bees' immune systems, directly decreasing their resistance to other environmental pressures. For this reason, we never place new hives in areas where there is an existing overpopulation of hives or a shortage of existing forage. To offset the environmental impact of hives, we also plant extensively, creating our own community gardens and encouraging businesses to sponsor local gardening groups and charities to plant the trees and bushes that supply the most fundamental elements of the honeybees' diet. A popular myth is that planting wildflower patches will save the honeybees; sadly, that's just not a reality.

So how does this all translate into the honey we produce? Crucially, we will never take a honey crop at the expense of our bees' welfare, harvesting only the surplus that the hive has produced above what it needs to overwinter as a strong, healthy colony. Neither will we treat our bees with anything except natural remedies.

Healthy bees feeding on a rich variety of natural forage produce delicious honey. Our job as artisan honey producers is to harvest and handle that product with great care, to preserve delicate natural flavours and important nutritional qualities. In the footsteps of artisan honey makers through the centuries, our honey is always sold 'raw'. Nothing is added or taken away. It is never subjected to heat above the natural hive temperature, or to blending, pressure-pumping, or microfiltering. These are just some of the disruptive processes used by commercial honey packers to produce cheap, commoditized 'supermarket' honeys with standardized colour and viscosity, but little, if any, food value.

The difference between our small-batch raw honeys and mass-produced commodity honeys is like the difference between rare, single estate coffee beans and a jar of freeze-dried instant coffee granules. It is all about provenance: our care for the environment, care for our bees, and care for our product creates the unique English honeys that so many consumers are now looking for. We are incredibly proud of our work and of our role within the artisan food community, collaborating with a wide range of fellow producers and sustainability initiatives. We also supply our honeys to craft brewers, bakers, fermentaries, and many other small businesses who, like us, value wholly natural ingredients of the highest possible quality. Raw honey is alive with difference – in colour, texture, flavour, and aromatics; it is always a glorious thing to put some onto your tongue and explore its complexities.

HELPING HONEYBEES

People constantly ask us what they can do to 'help the bees'. Our answer is always the same: plant meaningful forage for them and buy your honey direct from small, preferably local, producers to support their work. Local beekeeping societies everywhere are keen to connect customers with their members and foster a strong interest in bees and real honey.

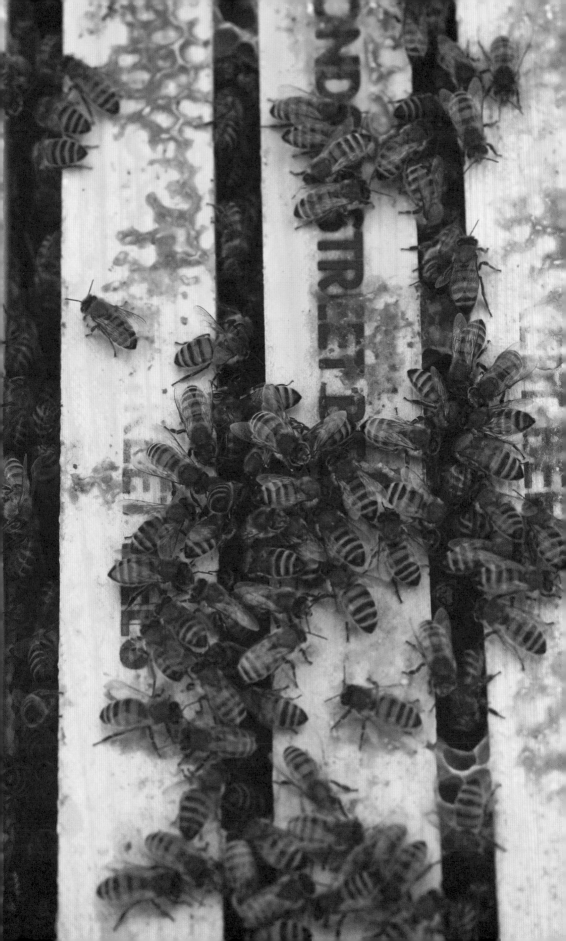

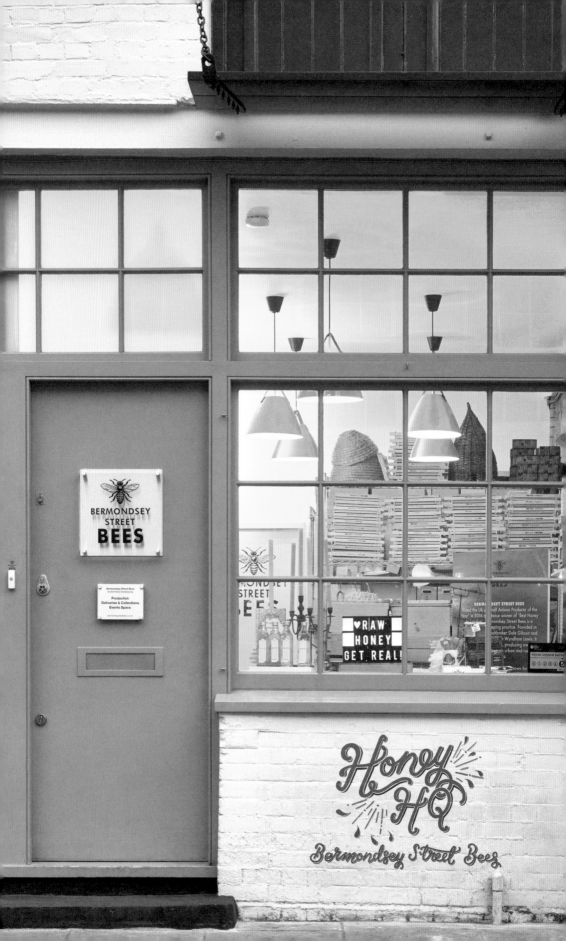

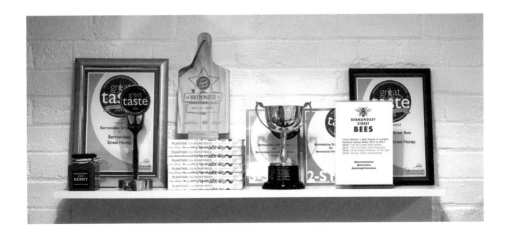

THE BEEKEEPING COMMUNITY

Our professional body, the Bee Farmers Association (BFA), represents the majority of commercial beekeepers in the UK – around 400 people (a shockingly small number given the economic value of pollination, honey, and other hive products). But no two members of the BFA have the same business profile. We are all beekeepers, but while some make a living supplying the big honey packers, others – like us – are very much at the craft end of honey production. And each of us has found our own way to build a business through offering a diverse range of products and services.

It has to be said that it is not easy to be a beekeeper, or to make a living from being one. It is very much a vocation. In our case, it was a second career for us both and we were happy to accept that luxuries we had taken for granted for many years would no longer be part of our lives. In effect, we are subsistence farmers. But we accept this happily, because everything that we now do is self-directed and has clear purpose.

> "We may be subsistence farmers, but we are also articulate activists on behalf of honeybees and their role in the wider ecology"

There are only two of us, but we work to make a difference on many different fronts, from selling the very best honey we can possibly make to putting bee-related policy considerations in front of powerful groups, from the Greater London Assembly to government ministers and PLC board members. Our first careers in the professional world still serve us well, and we are effective in creating opportunities to speak truth to power. We may be subsistence farmers, but we are also articulate activists on behalf of honeybees and their role in the wider ecology.

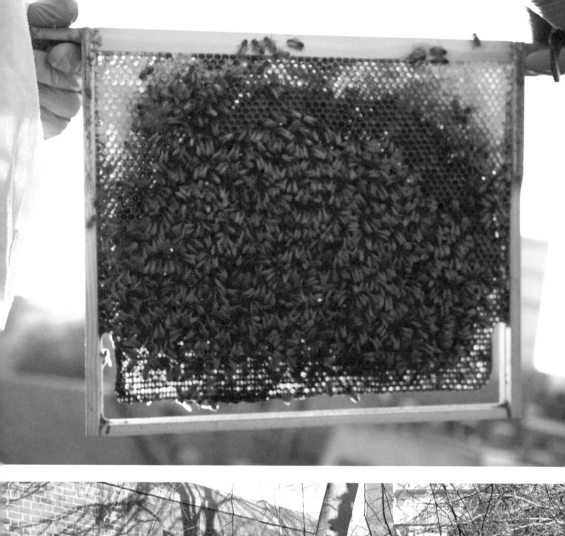

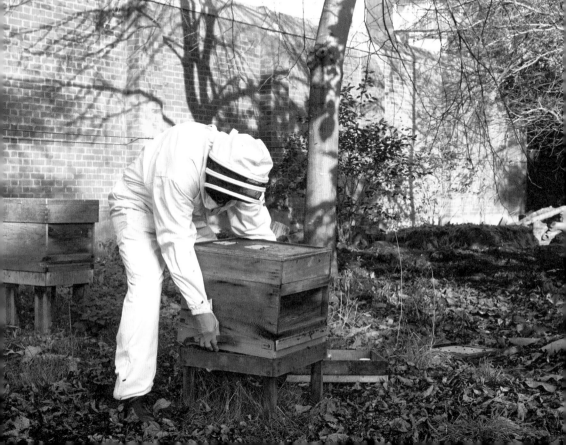

A BEEKEEPER'S CALENDAR

Day to day, we juggle a hectic schedule of managing eighty colonies across fourteen different urban and rural apiary sites, with our honey sales and deliveries, teaching and speaking appearances, collaborations with other food producers, writing reports for commercial clients and – when time allows – working on a second book. (Our first book, *Planting for Honeybees*, was published by Quadrille in 2018 in four languages and sells worldwide.)

In winter, when bees are quietly huddled in the hive, we have time at our desks to catch up with paperwork and plan new projects. As we move into very early spring, we will hope to see our bees flying on warmer days, signalling that the colony has survived the worst of winter; when we take our first look inside the hives by the end of February, we will know how successfully or not. It is a watch-and-wait game that repeats itself, year in, year out.

For six months of the year, from March to August, Dale is out from early morning to dusk every day visiting apiaries on a strict rota, monitoring their welfare. It is hard physical labour and it is relentless; you skip inspections at your peril, as hives can quickly be lost to disease or swarming. We also keep an anxious eye on the succession of flowering in each individual area, to reassure ourselves that the bees have plenty to feed their brood and themselves.

In August, we will assess what harvest is available to us and bring it into our production space. For the next three months, we will be spinning out honey whenever we have a spare moment, although we become increasingly busy dispatching honey and our other products (such as our honey-based bodycare products and beeswax candles) in the run-up to Christmas. Easter is another peak sales period.

DISTRIBUTION

On the sales front, we used to distribute honey through delis and grocers, and sell at food markets, but we are now pulling back from that. Selling in jars is costly in terms of overheads, especially when some retailers then mark it up by one hundred per cent. Equally, on our scale, there is no profit in mail order. But we have now become known as a specialist honey supplier to many of London's leading restaurants and hotels, with high-profile chefs, including Michel Roux Jr and Tom Kerridge, supporting our work. Working in this sector has led not only to higher sales volumes but also to some very progressive collaborations, showcasing sustainably produced raw honey as a primary ingredient in an incredible range of recipes. This is good news not just for us but for all artisan honey producers.

FROM HIVE TO JAR

01 Harvesting Generally, we take a harvest from the hives just once a year, in the late summer as the colony begins to prepare itself for the winter ahead. Leaving the hive with the honey that the bees need to overwinter safely, we harvest only their surplus production.

02 Uncapping the honeycomb The combs are brought back from the apiary into our production space to be spun out. Each wooden 'super' contains ten frames of honey, sealed with wax by the bees to preserve it. The first job is to uncap the honeycomb by piercing the seal on the hexagonal cells.

THE SUPER

The super, or honey box, is essentially a larder that is added to the hive setup as needed. The queen, brood, workers, and drones live in the brood box, which is the heart of the hive. When that is full of honey, the workers will look for other places to build comb and store honey, and will continue filling up supers as long as the nectar income is available from plants. At harvest time, we leave the bees all the honey they need to overwinter safely (around twenty kilograms per hive) and – if there is a surplus to take – we can remove supers without disturbing the colony.

03 Extraction As each frame in uncapped, it is placed into the honey extractor, carefully balancing the load. It is then spun out by centrifugal force and forms a waxy pool in the bottom of the drum. Emptied of honey, the spun-out combs will be returned to the hive from which they came.

04 First filtering The 'honey gate' (a porthole that can be opened to allow honey to flow out or locked to stop the honey going anywhere) at the bottom of the spinner is opened to allow the honey to flow into the bucket below, passing through a coarse stainless steel filter that removes beeswax.

05 Collecting wax Remaining beeswax fragments are saved and will be cleaned and recycled. Wax is widely used in industry, from the outer coatings of cheeses to textile production and lost-wax casting.

06 Second filtering Later, the honey is passed through a second filter to remove more wax. Although the filter looks superfine to the human eye, the mesh size comfortably allows pollen grains of all sizes to pass straight through with the honey.

07 Resting The honey rests in buckets at an ambient temperature to ripen. At no point in the honey production process should raw honey be subjected to heat in excess of the natural hive temperature (36 °C). Higher temperatures damage both its food value and its delicate flavours.

08 Packaging The honey is jarred by hand using UK-manufactured jars made from recycled glass. The honey gate is opened just enough to allow a manageable flow from the bucket into the jar, which sits on a set of commercial scales.

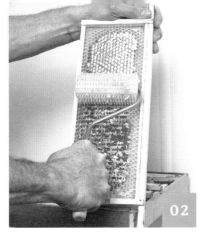

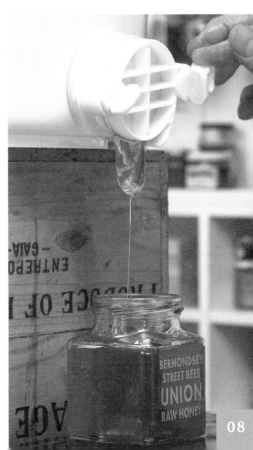

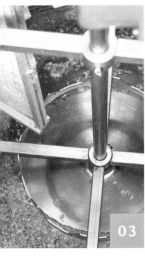

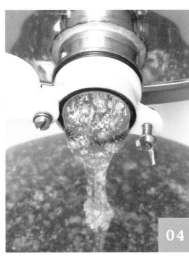

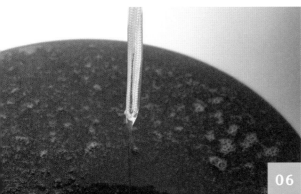

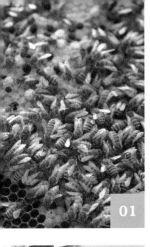

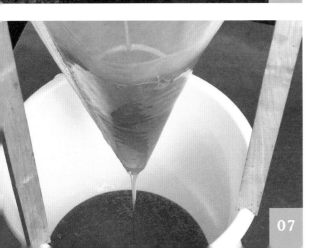

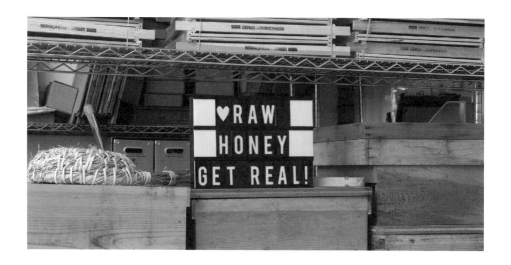

HONEY IN THE
TWENTY-FIRST CENTURY

Lack of forage, climate change, an ever-multiplying array of pests and diseases, the increasing frequency of hive thefts and numerous other pressures see many beekeepers shaking their heads over their long-term prospects.

Honey yields across the UK have fallen for decades, reflecting the continuous erosion of natural forage in town and country. In London, we contend with the densest hive population in Europe (hobby beekeeping has become super trendy) set against an annual loss of green space in Greater London equivalent to two-and-a-half times the area of Hyde Park.[11] In the countryside, the devastating impact of monoculture farming has led to the loss of a significant percentage of bees' natural foraging grounds since the 1930s.

The modern world can therefore be a profoundly hostile place for the honeybee, although the demand for honey continues to grow. This has led to honey being part of a very murky international trade and named as the third most adulterated foodstuff on earth, after wine and olive oil. Produced under dubious circumstances in countries that turn a blind eye to product purity and bee welfare, often trans-shipped and relabelled in more 'respectable' countries that legitimize access to world markets, blended and bulked out with sugars such as corn and rice syrup, super-heated, super-filtered, and processed to the point where it could be arguably said to be toxic, this so-called 'honey' ends up on supermarket shelves at bargain prices. Because that – apparently – is what the consumer demands.

Real honey is a luxury food. From the beginning, we made a conscious decision not to compete with the big-brand honey producers or to service the multiples. Instead we simply make and sell a premium product and educate consumers to understand the investment we make in that quality. Just like wine and olive oil, honey is an unpredictable annual harvest – it is very personal too, born of years of experience and physical labour. Time-intensive and expensive to produce, there is no 'halfway' process which straddles the old and new worlds. You either make good raw honey using the time-honoured methods or you sell out and produce a high-volume, low-cost commodity.

At ground level as UK honey producers we are subject to a raft of national and local regulations governing everything from how our honey is produced to how it is labelled and sold. There is particularly close focus on small producers like us rather than on the national honey brands, making us more likely to face attention from bodies such as Trading Standards and the Food Standards Authority. However, in the main, the regulations are fair and appropriate, and we feel that they make us better producers.

Running a honey business means lots of record-keeping and paperwork; our office is always flat-out with administration, sales, distribution, and front-of-house activities. Behind it all is the beekeeping itself and it is hard to find brain space to strategize and plan, especially in the hectic months between March and September when we often work eighteen-hour days without weekends. But we try to make time at least once a week to go out to breakfast together, taking our diaries with us for a catch-up ... But mainly to try to free up our minds to stay as creative as possible. Some of our very best ideas are worked out in the café across the road or in the car on road trips to visit distant hives. Luckily, our world of bees and beekeeping is both fascinating and beautiful, so social media works brilliantly for us too, and we maintain a high profile across several related accounts, snatching odd moments to post content and stay in touch with our customer base.

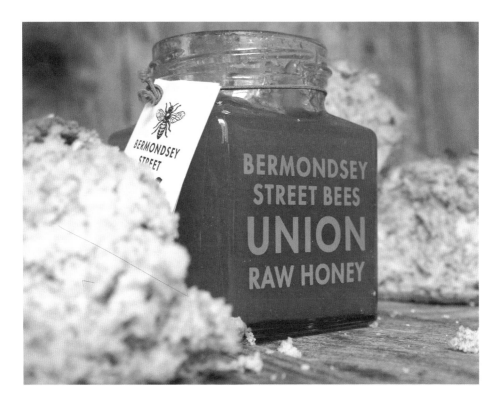

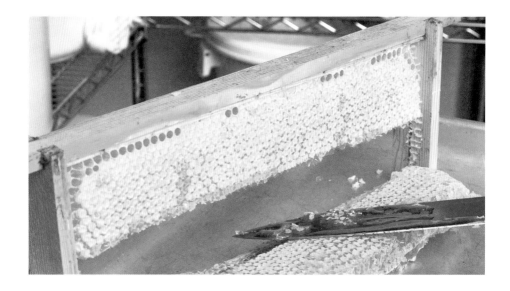

PRESERVING A HISTORIC CRAFT

Beekeeping is both an art and a science. It is also a journey of lifelong learning and most experienced beekeepers are generous with their time and their advice, investing in bringing newbies into the ranks.

There are no straight lines though and two sayings are worth relating: our own mentor John Chapple's quiet observation that 'bees don't read the same books we do' and the often-quoted 'if there are four beekeepers in a room, you'll have six different opinions'. Differences of opinion are the norm in beekeeping, but everyone finds their own route in the end. The mentorship system is therefore vital, not only to help beginners find their way but as a support network going forwards. It is also a very social world; beekeepers enjoy nothing more than hanging out with other beekeepers, to agree, disagree, talk shop, and exchange important information about the challenges we all face.

As experienced beekeepers ourselves, we maintain the long tradition of apprenticeships and mentoring, taking newer beekeepers with us through a year in the life of our bees and our business. It is time consuming, but it underlines the value we place on the direct transmission of knowledge, passing a historic craft down from hand to hand, with the addition of scientific know-how.

The golden days when beekeeping was a quiet, bucolic pastime are sadly now long gone. Today's beekeepers need to be equipped with a constantly updated armoury of knowledge, enabling them to weather a battery of threats – from the Varroa mite (the single most pernicious threat to honeybees) to countless other pests and diseases which have now reached UK shores. For this reason, we are firm believers in all beginners undertaking formal training and exams through the British Beekeeper's Association. Later too, as you become more experienced, because you should never stop learning – whether working towards high level awards such as Master Beekeeper or informally, by attending lectures and courses. The more that you invest in learning, the more that beekeeping will bring you, personally and professionally.

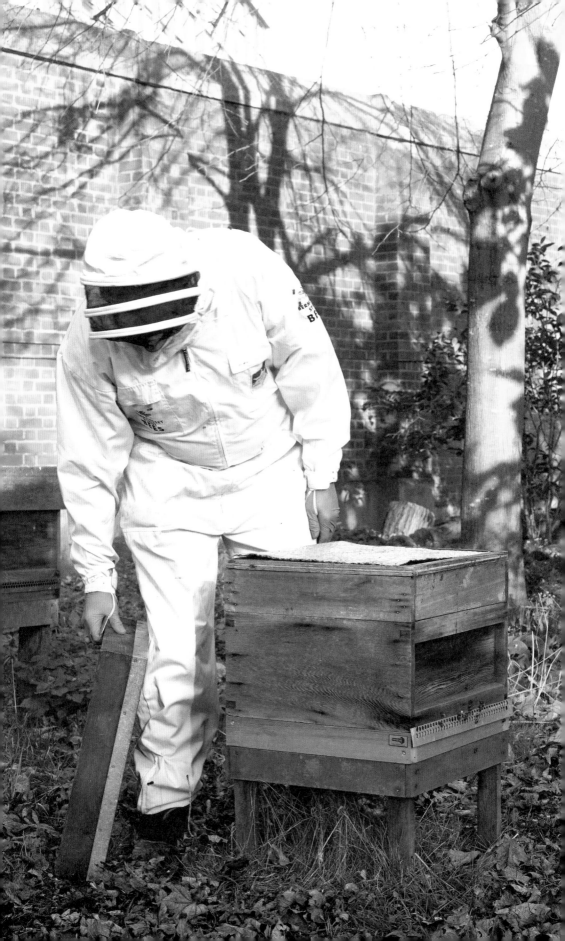

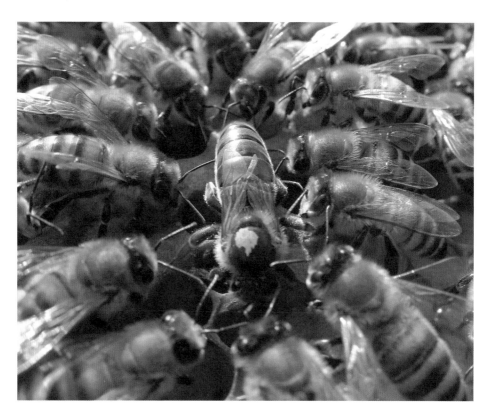

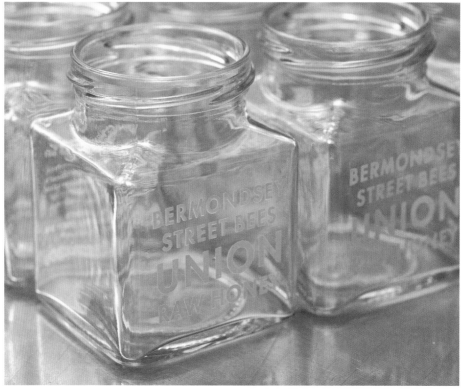

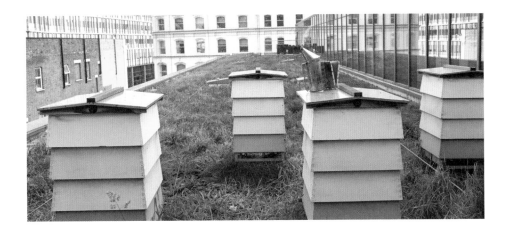

PROTECTING THE ENVIRONMENT

Another of our other founding philosophies is our commitment to conservation and minimal environmental impact. This extends through every level of the business, from planting forage for our honeybees to recycling all packaging that comes in to us. We use green energy to power the business, we employ locals, and we buy locally wherever possible; our English-made recycled glass jars come from under a mile away, as does the majority of our printing. Whenever possible, we do our local deliveries and beekeeping visits by bike. None of our honey is wasted either; our 'Salt & Honey Hand Scrub' was specifically developed to use the rich wax/honey residue which gets left behind in our cold-filtering process.

At every point of our work our business is utterly transparent, and we often invite people to come and see it close up, to learn more about what we do and how and why we do it. Through production room visits, talks, lectures, garden visits, bee experiences, and tutored honey tastings, we explain the eighty-million-year-old story of the honeybee, the extraordinary role which honey has played in cultures, ancient and modern, and the issues that face bees today. Hopefully too, we replace tired and lazy media myths about the honeybee with empowering facts.

"It is extraordinary how the world changes when you start to see it through the eyes of a bee"

In the end, our time and effort are directed to three things: caring for our bees, making exceptional honeys, and furthering people's understanding of the issues at stake. It is hard work and will never make us rich. But it's easy to offset that against the joys of living and working with one of nature's most complex social creatures. Our days revolve around their life cycle and we have learned to narrow our gaze from macro to micro. It is extraordinary how the world changes when you start to see it through the eyes of a bee.

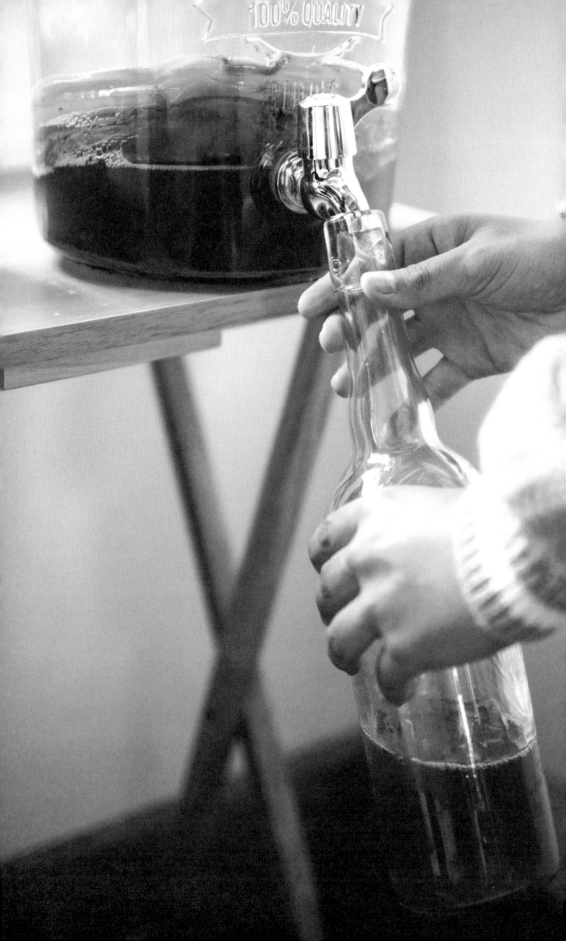

APPLE CIDER VINEGAR

Vinegars have been made and valued by humankind for thousands of years. They can be crafted from a variety of natural foods as long as the original ingredients have a high sugar content. Apple cider vinegar is a natural by-product of the apple cider-making process and is created when apple cider is left to ferment. In its raw, unfiltered, and unpasteurized state, it can make a characterful drink or can be applied externally as a product. It is said to have many potential health benefits, beauty benefits, and skin-soothing properties.

"Seeing the fruits of these ancient trees being turned into a modern-day elixir is amazing"

William Chase, Willy's ACV

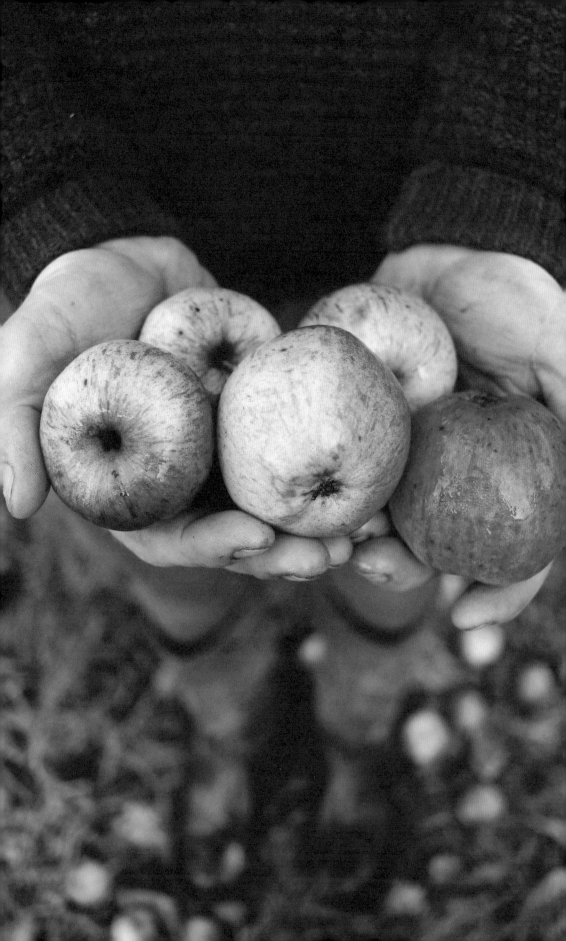

WILLY'S ACV

WILLIAM CHASE

Herefordshire, UK | willysacv.com

I live and breathe the magic of the county I live in. It is where I was born, where I am raising my family, and where I have built my businesses. Herefordshire is unspoilt, underdeveloped, and natural. The soil is red and fruitful and the views are serene. I enjoy being here, making brands with pedigree from the fruit of this amazing area. I have been a potato farmer for a large part of my life, until landing on the idea to make characterful crunchy crisps in 2002 with Tyrrells, and then single-estate spirits with Chase Distillery in 2008. Little did I know, however, that moving to my current home (Laddin Farm, Little Marcle) in 2005 would open up a third and the most exciting of ventures using apples from the 200 acres of beautiful old orchards surrounding my house. Being here is like being in an untouched natural biome. The original trees have remained unaffected by modern-day farming practices and the natural way we maintain the land results in the most incredible natural diversity. The place sings.

While the distillery sales continued to grow nicely, an awareness that people were searching for an altogether more mindful approach to life – from what they consume to how they treat the environment – meant that I started seeing the apple crop around the farm in a new light. Here in the orchards was the means to make one of nature's most potent, natural remedies: apple cider vinegar. The process to make it was also only one step further on from my existing process at the distillery. I leave the apple cider vinegar raw and unfiltered, so the amazing 'mother culture' – a colony of probiotic bacteria that forms at the final fermentation stage – is alive and full of goodness in this remarkable natural remedy.

AN ERA OF MINDFUL CONSUMPTION

I believe a large section of society is now extremely mindful of the food and drink they consume and will actively choose brands that complement their moral conscience about ethical supply, fair process, health and wellness, and environmental impact. My apple cider vinegar is sustainable because from apple to bottle, I am controlling the whole process, using very few food miles. I grow my own apples in a natural, sustainable way in Herefordshire. Other ingredients are sourced locally where possible. For example, Willy's Natural Energy Drink is made of five clean, all-natural ingredients: apple cider vinegar, green tea kombucha (both fermented at the farm), water (drawn from a source beneath the orchards), apple juice (from a neighbouring supplier), and ginger. I have a small team that farms the orchards and handles the process of pressing, fermenting, bottling, and selling the product. We pack our apple cider vinegar in glass bottles and our range of fermented drinks is packed in recyclable aluminium cans. Our labels are made of paper and our outer boxes are made of cardboard. We also recycle any waste apple pulp via our anaerobic digester. The fertilizer produced from this is then ploughed back into the orchards. We handle everything ourselves, sharing it out between the team of eleven growing, fermenting, bottling, selling, and marketing. We even design all our packaging ourselves.

"Small acts can collectively lead to great benefits, like trying to buy a percentage of your shopping from local independents"

CONSCIOUS SPENDING

There is an increasing awareness of the ethical and health benefits of locally sourced food and drink; however, so much more can be done to educate people about the ethics of supporting local producers and retailers. Small acts can collectively lead to great benefits, like trying to buy a percentage of your shopping from local independents, or buying brands that have been produced within the locality, whether that is an online purchase directly from them or via a store.

I am always hugely respectful of specialist independents that bring many of these small producers' dreams to life. Local farm shops have helped me share the fruits of my craft with local consumers and continue to be the backbone of my success. Like loyal friends, they have bought into my story and supported me through each of my chapters. Behind each small brand or retailer is an incredibly dedicated and passionate group of people.

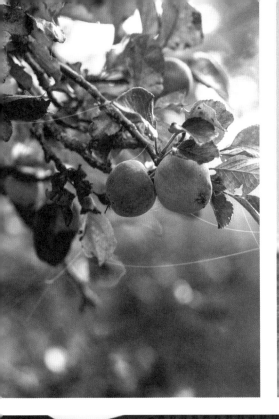
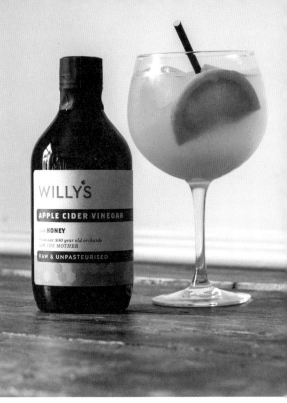
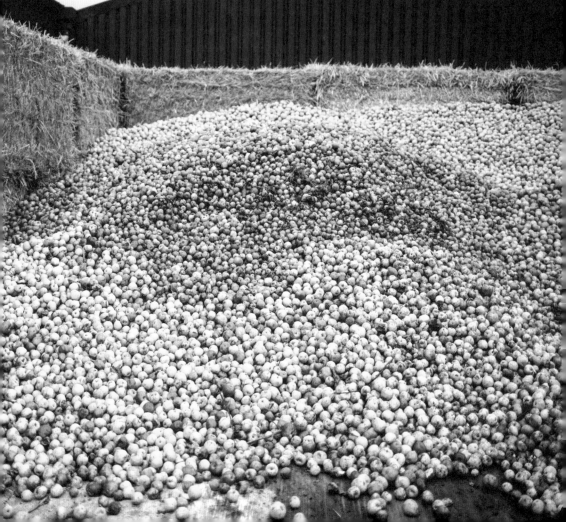

A NATURAL REMEDY

I have travelled far and wide to learn all about the craft of making each and every one of my brands. Since turning my attention to apples, I have been intrigued by the history of natural remedies. I am especially curious as my Chase family ancestors were apothecaries to King Charles II in the 1660s, so some could say it is in my genes to work with nature and all her amazing healing properties. It fascinates me how people have used fermentation for centuries and how, when harvested and cultivated in a safe and stable way, friendly bacteria in food and drink can not only heal, but also help us maintain ongoing wellness. From Roman times, apple cider vinegar has been used for strength, wellness, and healing. A blend of water and vinegar called 'posca' was sold in the streets that was believed would make you strong, versus wine, which made you drunk, or in Latin: *Posca fortem, vinum ebrium facit.*

"I aim to make a tried-and-trusted product that is honest at heart and not exposed to any artificial processes"

Seeing the fruits of these ancient trees being turned into a modern-day elixir is amazing. It is all about the mother culture: she was here, under my nose for years and now she is alive in every bottle and working her magic. Apple cider vinegar is wonderfully versatile in terms of how you consume it. I take a daily dose of apple cider vinegar mixed with beetroot juice, whereas my wife enjoys it with water and some slices of ginger and lemon. I have lost weight, reduced my cholesterol, and also sleep better since I have started my daily dose. I would recommend not drinking it straight though!

I aim to make a tried-and-trusted product that is honest at heart and not exposed to any artificial processes. It is full of probiotic goodness that has so many claimed health benefits – from balancing pH in the gut, to helping regulate blood sugar levels and reduce cholesterol. It is a one hundred per

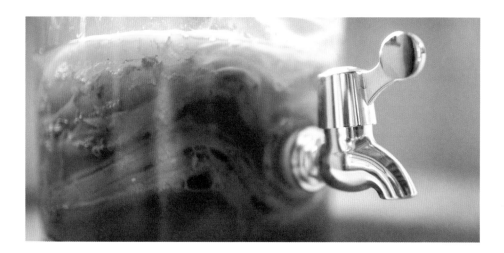

cent natural remedy. To support this, I aspire to be a pioneer in 'probiotic' farming, farming the land without a hint of chemicals or artificial fertilizers to create the most natural, symbiotic balance within the orchards.

Probiotic farming uses a variety of techniques, including the use of natural effective microorganisms, fermentation, and composting to create healthier crop yields without disrupting the natural cycle around the trees. We have a programme to entice beneficial predator insects like ladybirds, lacewings, hoverflies, and earwigs to naturally keep the aphid count low rather than using pesticides. The best way to attract them is with wildflowers and herbs, which we plant in spring. We also give them a varied home in our fields in the form of bug hotels. Small birds are another option for natural pest control – particularly for codling moths, a pest in the apple world – so we try to help the birds feel at home in our orchard by introducing a feeding area, for example. The apples then sourced from these orchards are fermented into apple cider vinegar with help from our very own unique mother culture, creating a probiotic closed loop – from soil to the finished natural, fermented ACV.

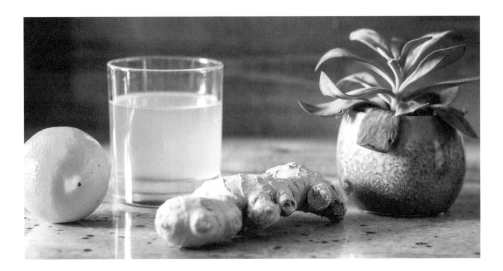

A STORY TO BE TOLD

The greatest story of all lies with 'The Mother' in my apple cider vinegar. She is of the orchards, literally. She is present in the pips and stalks, the bark, and the boughs of the apple trees surrounding the farm. During the process of making apple cider vinegar, she forms her colonies of probiotic, gut-friendly bacteria in each batch, with a small part of the farm's history continuously being passed through the apple cider vinegar into each bottle. You will see her alive and floating in the bottles – sometimes as small particles, other times as a cobwebby mass. Many mass-manufacture apple cider vinegar producers remove the culture to avoid the cloudy appearance. The cloudiness is where the goodness lies, however, so don't ever be afraid of her. She is the apple of our eye and the secret to the success of Willy's Apple Cider Vinegar.

BEHIND THE SCENES

We own 200 acres of pristine apple orchards in Herefordshire, where we grow forty-eight apple varieties – including several old heritage varieties. In autumn, the apples drop naturally and are left to rest to allow the sugars to mature and consequently the taste to intensify.

A special apple harvest tractor with rollers gently scoops the apples from between the trees before they're sent to be pressed.

Yeast is added to the pressed apple juice to break down the natural sugars and turn it into a delicious bittersweet cider. Then, in a special tank called an acetator, the combination of Herefordshire fresh air and the 'mother culture' slowly turns the cider into craft ACV.

Finally, the apple cider vinegar is transferred to oak casks to rest and mature in taste and body.

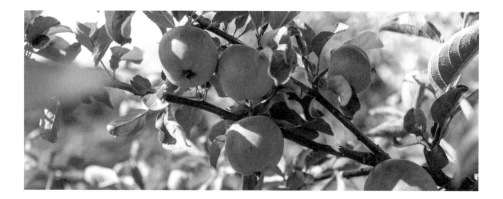

A TYPICAL DAY

My place of work is my home. I have converted a small barn on site at Laddin Farm from which we run the customer services, sales, marketing, and finance. A typical day would involve getting up around 5.00 am and prioritizing tasks for the day, from the farm to finance. I am an early bird and find my inspiration flows first thing. I split my time with the team in the office and on site where we ferment and bottle. I am happiest in Herefordshire, but I enjoy travelling to London and beyond to research new ideas at trade shows such as Expo West Wellness show in the USA or Speciality & Fine Food Show in Singapore. I love to meet with like-minded producers and believe in sharing a few secrets in return for new knowledge and expertise. Every day is a new opportunity to learn.

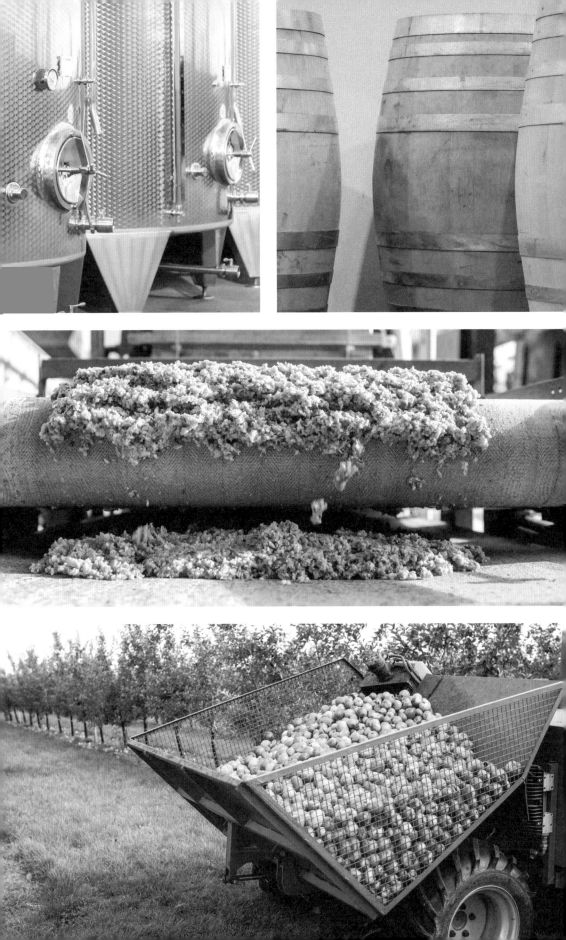

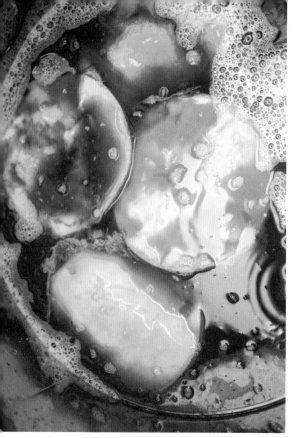

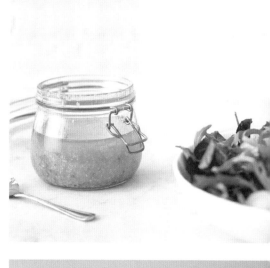

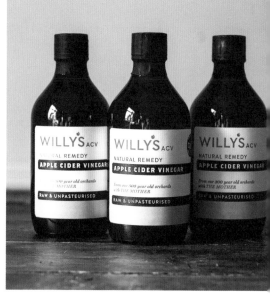

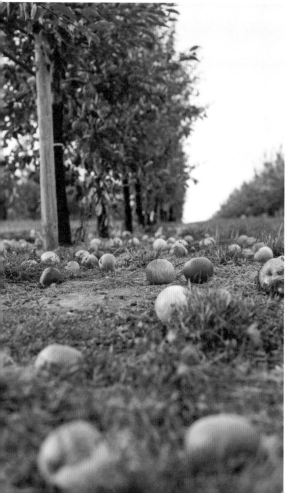

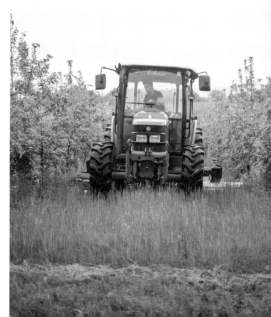

NURTURING A BUSINESS

We are growing in sales each month as we spread the word about the benefits of apple cider vinegar. When you are a small brand with a relatively new concept, you have got to make as much noise as possible on a small budget, so each day needs to be a busy day. At the time of writing, we have only been selling in earnest for about a year and a half so it is difficult to see a trend yet. However, I anticipate a peak in the new year as people use it as a cleansing natural remedy and again in summer when it can be used as a dressing in salads.

Most of our sales are through small independent retailers, from places like Bayley & Sage and John Bell & Croyden in London to amazing specialist delis and family farm shops up and down the country. They are the lifeblood of the business. Specialist distributors like Hider, Suma, and Marigold can help you reach some stores that operate a strict supply chain. We sell nationally through customers like Waitrose, and are starting to build up our international sales in neighbouring European markets. We now also have a subscription scheme (the Willy's Wellness Box) to help converts receive a box of our products, a selection of recipes, and also a gift from like-minded sustainable brands each month.

We made contact and built relationships with retailers by sending out thousands of samples. A big percentage of our spend goes towards sending samples to potential customers so they trial the product. We work with food groups such as the Guild of Fine Food and the Farm Retail Association (formerly FARMA) to build our database of independent retailers; then it is a case of picking up the phone or visiting in person to develop relationships. These outlets are not necessarily swayed by the size of your following on social media – they will buy on pedigree, story, and passion for the brand. We also exhibit at trade shows such as the Farm Shop & Deli Show and the Natural & Organic Products Europe Show to recruit new customers, plus run samplings with our biggest independent retailers. In the case of the latter, a dedicated member of the Willy's team runs samplings at the customer's premises during a weekend. This can generate an uplift of up to ten times the number of sales and allows us to educate consumers about the befits of the product firsthand, at no extra cost to the retailer.

GRANTS AND FUNDING

It can be very worthwhile looking into grants and funding opportunities in your local area. We received a Rural Development Grant in 2018 to support the cost of purchasing further apple cider vinegar production equipment. We discovered this grant through research with help from the local chamber of commerce business team. We also receive support from the Marches Local Education Provider, supporting us with the provision of training, as well as funding from the Education & Skills Funding Agency.

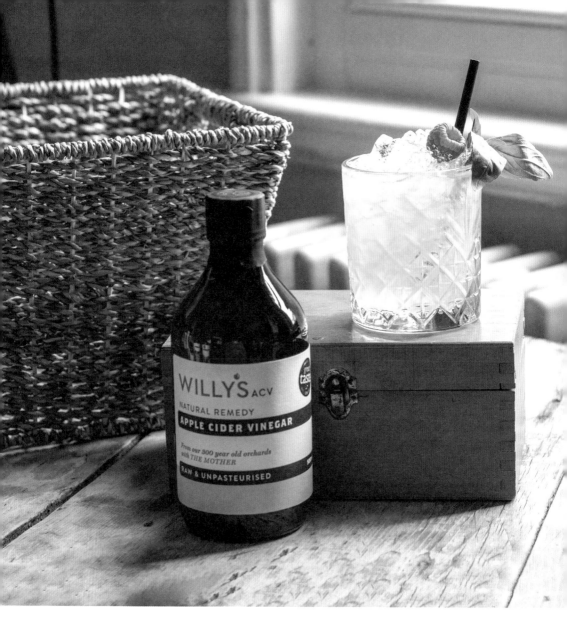

THE POWER OF BRANDING

I believe that marketing boils down to simple, great communication. As well as excellent quality and memorable packaging, a great story sells a brand. The best brands have an emotional connection with their customers and serve a true purpose in their life by either solving a need or creating a moment of delight in their daily life. Brand magic is such an amazing thing. I believe the magic in the Willy's brand is in the quality of our mother culture, which is unique to my orchards.

Willy's is a social brand. We are approachable and friendly so, while our sales are still relatively small, we have a significant following of fans across social media. It is an extremely important conduit for all the amazing testimonials we receive from our followers. Social media allows our followers to share experiences and recipes, from showing the vinegar's potential in aiding weight loss to

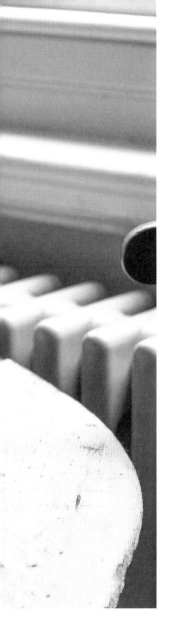

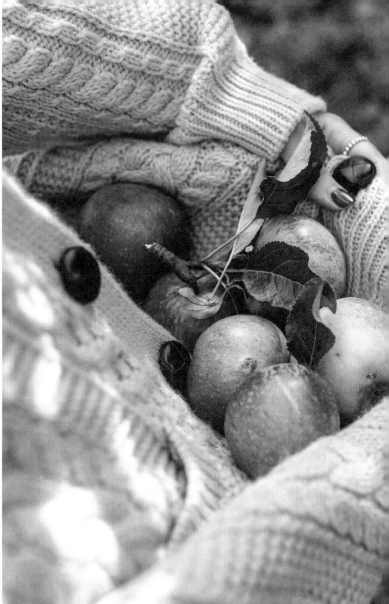

relieving digestion issues. We are an extremely transparent brand too; based on a farm in the heart of Herefordshire, we are constantly sharing images of daily life at the farm. It is real and the source of beautiful social media fodder.

DISCOVER AND BE YOUR BRAND
Find your brand magic – from the process to the people. Define what will make you stand out from the crowd and then make it your single-minded focus. Live and breathe it. It is going to be such a lot of hard work but seeing a brand idea turn into a product on a shelf and comments on social media is infectious.

INTEGRATING TRADITION
WITH INNOVATION

With the ease at which we can gather information and make connections since the launch of smartphones, I believe the world is truly in our palm 24/7. I am insanely curious, so I spend some part of each day looking at trends and innovation from all corners of the globe. I never imagined I would evolve from one day being a humble potato farmer to now farming live cultures to help gut health.

Any successful brand should strive to be at the forefront of innovation, but you can mix tradition with cutting-edge technology to achieve amazing results. Now that sales are growing steadily, I recently invested in a fantastic piece of equipment from Germany that allows me to produce apple cider vinegar (and also fermented drinks like kombucha) in a safe, stable, and consistent way. It is a state-of-the-art bespoke piece of equipment, but I still place my apple cider vinegar in oak casks at the end of the process to give it a beautiful rounded taste.

I am not fazed by bigger brands or supermarkets. The innovation is happening in the speciality market. Retailers often look to the smaller independent stores for the latest revolutionary, trend-setting brands. I think consumers deserve to be able to buy good brands online or nationally from a range of outlets, but I also think small producers deserve respect. It is nice to see a few bigger retailers now setting up incubator programmes to nurture entrepreneurial new brands, with lots of support to help get them going. While artisan small-batch methods can evolve into scaled-up manufacturing, I very much think that retaining the magic of a brand – whether small or large – lies in attitude and behaviour. I am a great believer in being modest and humble, respecting your roots and always staying true to the brand's values and ethos.

KEEP AN EYE ON TRENDS

As a brand owner, preparing yourself for fluctuations in consumer trends is also a big watch-out. Interestingly, in Herefordshire, there is a boom and bust on the cider apple front. Bittersweet apples have fallen out of favour as consumers swap to fruity, sweet ciders versus traditional variants, meaning acres of bittersweet orchards have been bulldozed over the last five years. I am fortunate, however, that bittersweet apples are the main ingredient in apple cider vinegar, so while the trend for natural remedies grows, I am able to rescue acres of land to grow against an all-together healthier side to the apple trend.

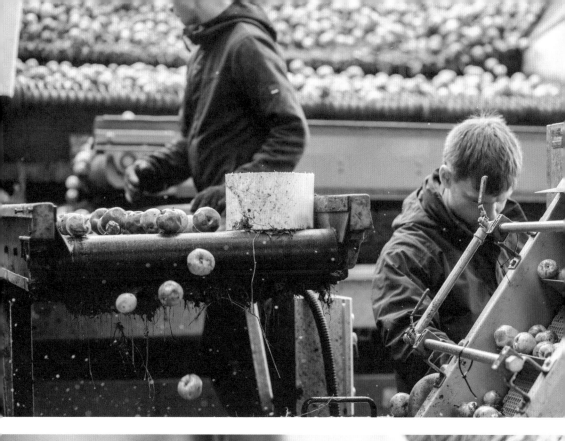

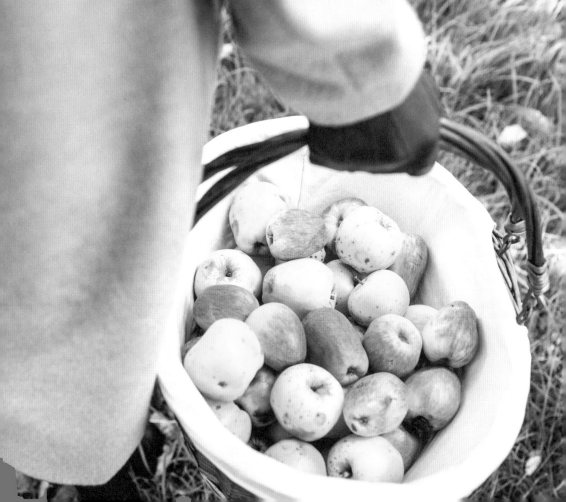

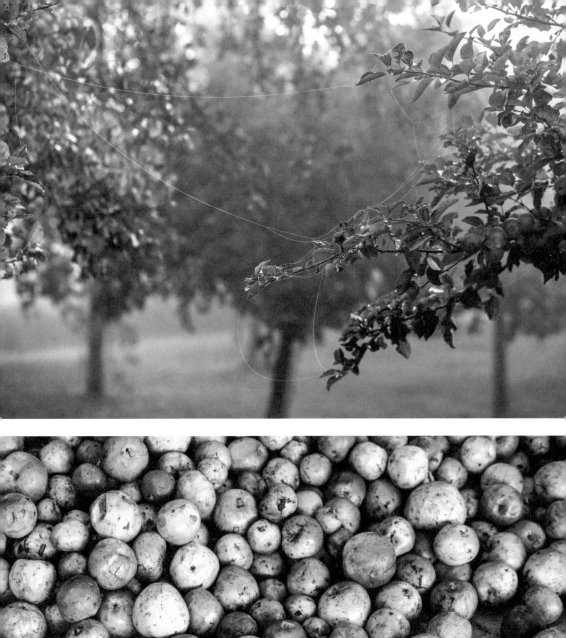
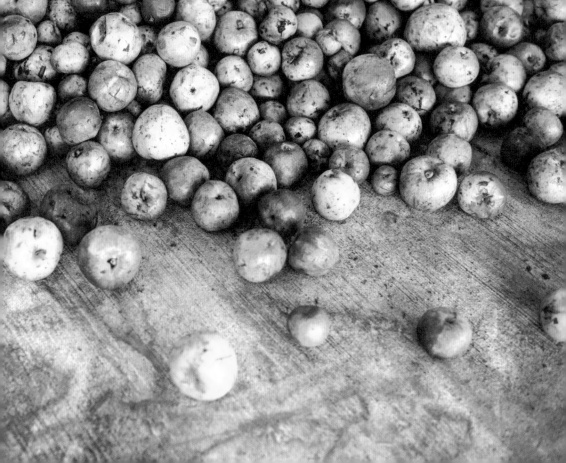

LOOKING TO THE FUTURE

Farming is in my blood. My mother and father farmed cattle and turkey as well as perry pears, cider apples, and potatoes here in Herefordshire. My world has been dictated by the seasons. From a young age, I have been involved with nurturing the land around me for the purpose of making a living, so naturally I am always curious and inquisitive about what I can grow and make in the fields within my county. In terms of the next generation, I am fortunate to have four sons. The oldest, Harry, has continued to farm in Herefordshire, growing potatoes for both Tyrrells Crisps and Chase Distillery. James has forged a career as a talented marketeer, and is now based in the USA shaping the future of the Chase Distillery brand there. It is hard to tell what direction my youngest two, Austin and Thomas (ten and eight), will take. I hope they share my curiosity and passion for creating something special from scratch, regardless of what it is.

Working with a raw natural crop, you are always at the mercy of Mother Nature. However, I am fortunate that in Herefordshire the land lends itself perfectly to growing cider apples, so continuity of the crop is protected to a great degree. My own orchards have survived for 300 years, so I am hoping I will get a fair few years out of these beautiful trees yet.

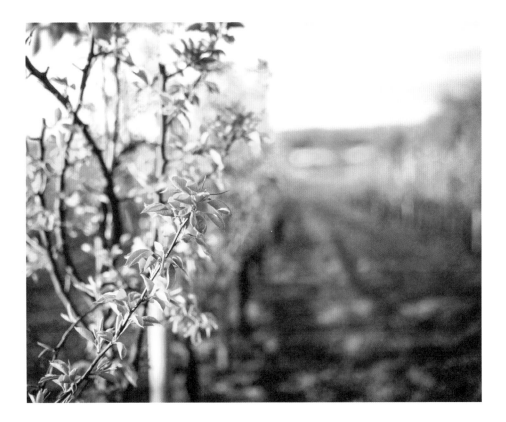

RESPONSIBLE SOURCING

It is not always possible for food artisans to grow their own ingredients. Sometimes they need to be sourced, and sourced ethically. Most of us are familiar with the concept of fair trade; in this section Beau Cacao demonstrate how they take this one step further through direct trade – building a rapport with farmers directly to ensure farmer and buyer benefit from the relationship without potential limitations that can be found in fair trade practices. The Authentic Bread Company are another business who strive to ensure their products are made from ethically sound ingredients, ensuring their packaging helps protect their integrity. Meanwhile, our coffee makers, Brandon and Kelleigh, are fortunate enough to be able to grow their own beans but highlight that this needs to be done at a responsible scale. They also demonstrate the importance of sharing their experience with other coffee farmers in the region in order to help other people work sustainably.

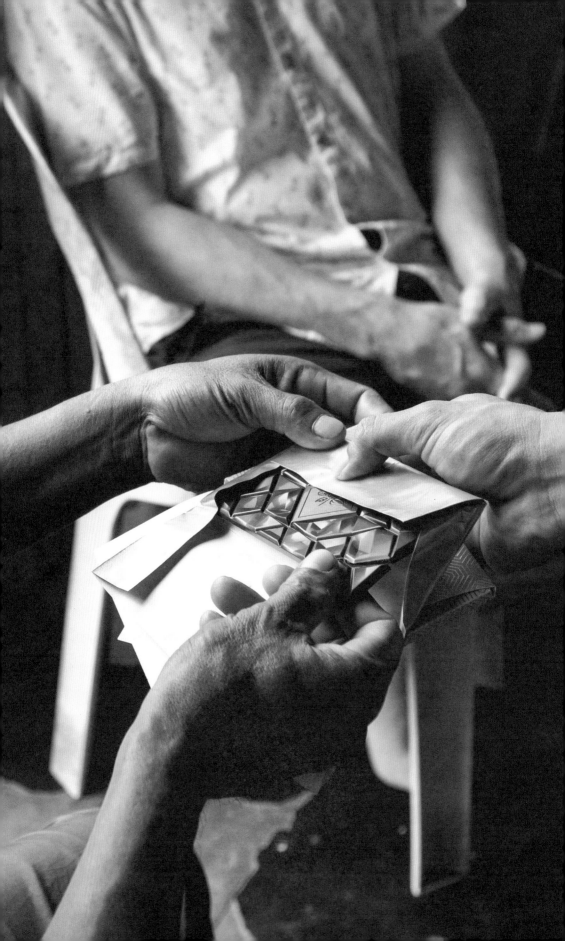

CHOCOLATE

Chocolate has a rich and enduring history. Served as a hot drink by the Mayans and a cold, spicy drink by the Aztecs, it has prevailed as a luxurious part of many people's diet. It is made from beans from the cacao tree, which belongs to the *Theobroma* genus – literally translated as 'food of the gods'.

Industrialization meant that chocolate recipes could be processed, set in moulds, and solidified in bars to form the kind of chocolate experience all of us know and love today. However, the fast-paced, mass-manufactured, mass-marketed chocolate industry does not always produce the highest quality and is not the only option. Artisan producers are fighting back and sourcing single-origin cocoa beans from individual farmers and creating and designing elegantly tailored craft chocolate. Enjoyed in this way, chocolate has come full circle and is once again a sought-after, luxury treat.

"Joy and happiness radiate with chocolate;
it makes people happy, it paints smiles,
it can mean the world to someone"

Bo San Cheung & Thomas Delcour, Beau Cacao

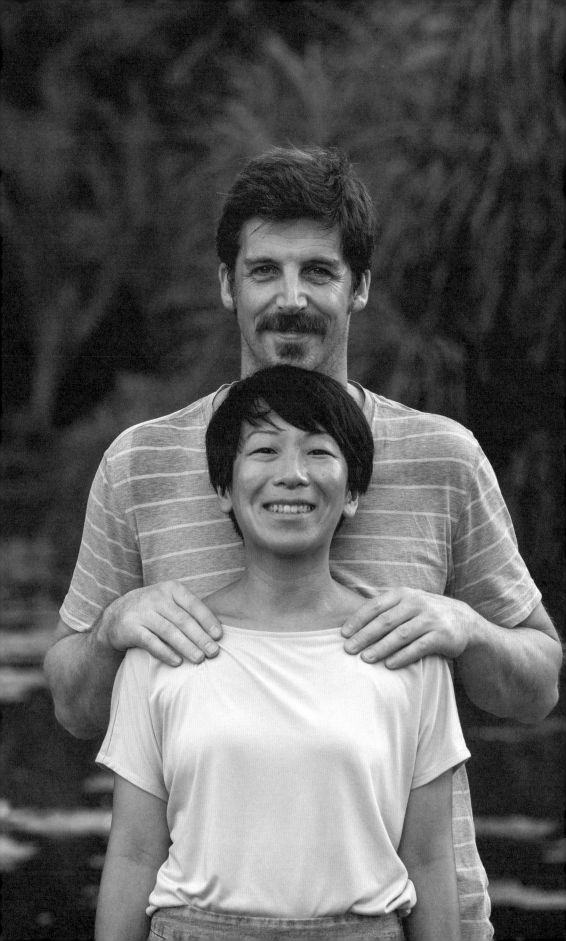

BEAU CACAO

BO SAN CHEUNG & THOMAS DELCOUR

Briançon, France | beaucacao.com

Realizing what is behind a chocolate bar felt like an untold fairy tale, and it all started when we met across the world in New Zealand. Our love for different continents and cultures kept us on the road for a few years after we met, and during this time we developed a huge interest in the origins of our food and the story behind each ingredient. Along this culinary journey we discovered that chocolate would be a part of our lives; learning that it is from a fruit was fascinating, and even more exciting was discovering that we could produce chocolate on a small scale – so small that we could even make it at home!

But we didn't want to make just any chocolate: we wanted it to serve a purpose for people and our planet, and to understand how to achieve this was to educate ourselves, step by step. We first learned theoretically – how to make chocolate and the science behind it, what machines to use and how to use them, and the history of cacao and where it grows. We also needed to understand the business side – the local and global markets, how to build a brand, how to create bespoke packaging, and which printing methods to use. In addition to these elements, one of the most challenging components of planning our project was considering how we would convey the message of what real chocolate is and how we appreciate its true value. We looked at the map of chocolate, where the cacao grew, and asked ourselves why no one made craft chocolate from Malaysian cocoa beans. That is when we explored plantations across Sarawak and Sabah, Borneo Island.

OUR VALUES

Stepping into the world of chocolate changed us as people. It raised our awareness of consumption and its impact on the planet, and from there on, we wanted to be part of the change that is happening today by being the change we would like to see. Our eyes opened to the way we consume food globally, and dedicating our lives to chocolate meant immersing ourselves in it and ensuring that every decision we make is made consciously. The connection between people and food is often lost, and for that reason we want to ensure that people know that the chocolate bar they are about to eat was made from cacao beans from farmers we have met.

There are four core values that motivate us daily in our personal and professional lives: ecological sustainability, health, animal welfare, and social welfare. We reject the modern mass-market approach to making chocolate. We create a direct link between you as the consumer and the cacao farmers and we are one hundred per cent committed to becoming a socially, environmentally responsible, and sustainable company. We are, however, aware that by creating a consumer product we harm our planet through the use of resources in production, so we are working hard to minimize this impact. For example, we do not use any animal products in our chocolate such as dairy and we consider our sources of energy very carefully. We are very lucky to set up in the beautiful city of Briançon, which has its own electricity supplied by a small hydraulic dam managed locally.

Our aim is to become part of the B-Corporation community (find out more on p. 272), which offers an incredibly useful framework through which to guide companies toward good environmental and social practices. We try to bring responsibility into our decision-making every day, and value the three Ps, in the following order: planet, people, profit. This is our biggest strength against the mass-market manufacturers who often do the exact opposite of those three Ps. If everybody supports companies with these values, we will be able to influence the big manufacturers to make a radical change to follow these values.

With the 'slow food movement', consumers are bringing more curiosity to the table and people are demanding more transparency from brands. They want to know how things are made, where it comes from, and the stories behind each product. This movement allows us small makers to meet those demands freely and easily, and it also helps people make a better, conscious decision that aligns with their own beliefs. Making things cheaply means someone else is paying the price, and it is often the ones at the beginning of the chain – in our industry it is the cacao farmers. Purchasing single-origin, fairly traded chocolate – or any ethically sourced or produced food – is a chance for everyone to get together and make an important change to their buying habits. Every pound, euro, or dollar you spend is a vote for a better ecosystem.

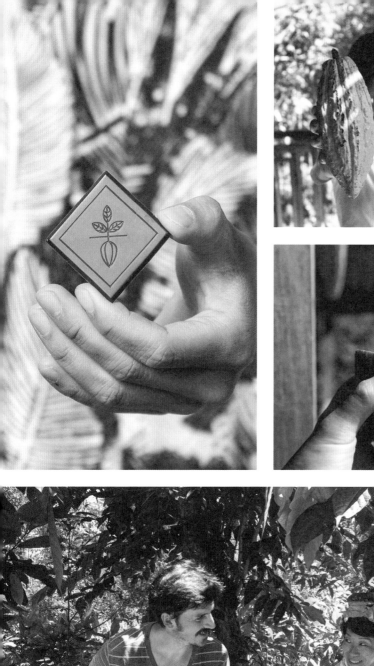
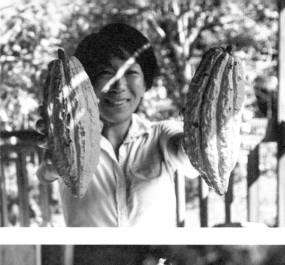
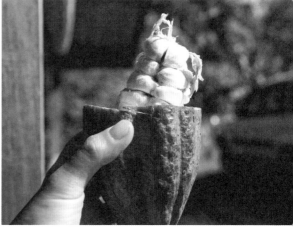
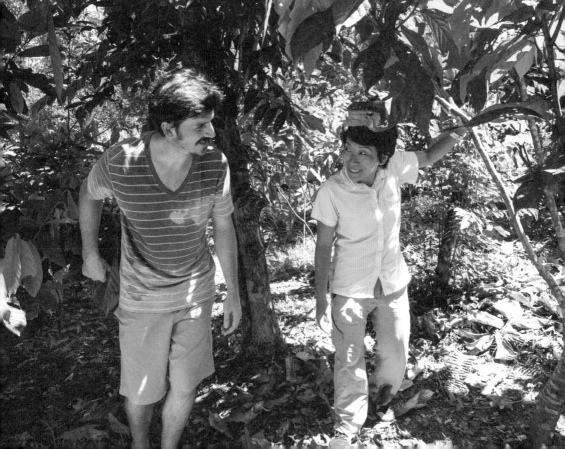

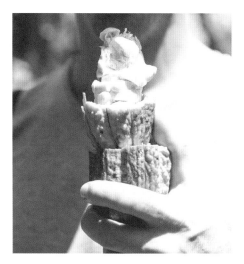

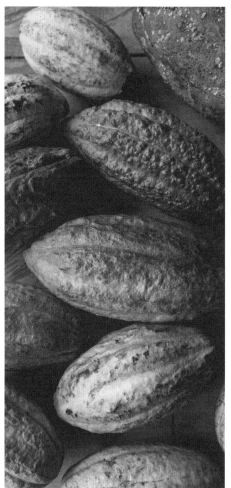

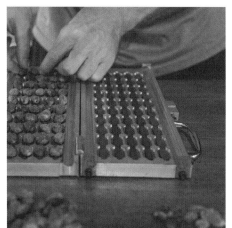

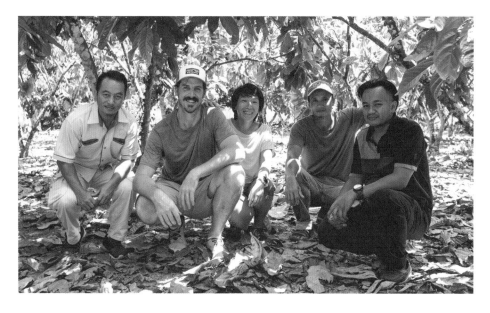

THE FARMERS

We built our brand hoping to change the way people think about chocolate and this meant we needed to build our foundations and start where the seeds grow into trees. Meeting farmers is part of our process, and because we are micro-scale it made sense to focus on one country, in this case Malaysia. Purely focusing on one country allows us to better understand our product offering, and have a better relationship with the people behind each of our ingredients, recognize their hard work, ensure they are paid correctly, and constantly improve what we do together. With this approach we go beyond fair trade and work with a direct trade ethos. We know exactly where the beans grow and who they have been grown by.

> "It is crucial that we tell the farmers' stories and our story ... not to enrich one person, but to sustain the entire chain"

We admire the people who grow these beautiful cacao trees. They are an integral part of the story of chocolate, and without their hard work there is no chocolate, as it is certainly a challenge to maintain a cacao plantation. The trees only grow twenty degrees north and south of the equator and they can grow on flat or varied gradients of terrain; it generally needs to be hot and humid. Visiting the trees very early in the morning or late afternoon is best in order to avoid the burning sun! It is crucial that we tell the farmers' stories and our story for a greater understanding that a product made with absolute adoration in each and every process is necessary – not to enrich one person, but to sustain the entire chain. This then gives each person the opportunity to make a living from what they love doing.

We are working with farmers to build long-term relationships and secure a sustainable supply of high-quality cacao. They truly inspire us with their beautifully maintained trees that bear the most colourful fruit you have ever seen. At the time of writing, we as a business are still very small scale, but when we do make a profit, it will be reinvested not only into our production line but also into the farms to improve the farmers' working conditions or to help them move towards more ecological practices, such as moving beyond monoculture to more agroforestry approaches.[12]

It is so important to pay the farmers well to encourage them to work for quality and not quantity. It also encourages the younger generation to be interested in farming, and to take pride in this incredible industry, knowing that it truly matters to the masses. We need to make sure farmers can thrive through their hard work as anyone should be able to, and show this next generation that there is a future in cacao so that they will be able to protect and impact positively on their local environment. For example, cacao trees come from under the jungle, so they grow and thrive very well under the forest. It can therefore be a very beneficial crop to grow to protect the forest and the animals while at the same time benefiting the people.

FROM BEAN TO BAR

SEEDS, BEANS, HUSKS & NIBS

When the cacao tree bears the fruit (cacao pod), which can come in various shapes and sizes, the farmers empty these pods. The pods are filled with a delicious pulp that surrounds the seeds (this pulp can be consumed, but you have to be careful not to bite into the seeds as they are extremely bitter at this point!), and it is these seeds that will be used to create the chocolate. The seeds are fermented and dried in the sun. When dried they are edible and ready for us to work with. At this stage we start to call them 'beans'.

A bean is composed of three parts: the seed coat, the kernel, and a germ. During the fermentation process, the germ and the seed coat are killed. Afterwards, we call the seed coat a 'husk'. During the roasting process, the kernel dries and becomes very brittle. When the roasting process is finished and we crack the kernel, its pieces are called nibs.

01 Sorting After the beans have been harvested and fermented, they need to be dried to stop them from fermenting any further. The beans are dried outside on large surfaces that are exposed to all sorts of things. Our very first job is to sort through the beans and find anything unwanted, from twigs to rope. We also discard small, odd-shaped, and defective beans as these make it difficult to crack and winnow later on in the process.

02 Roasting As a young, two-person company, we roast in micro-batches. It is affordable for us to roast in a standard-sized rotisserie oven, which allows us to control and evenly roast every batch. For each estate we go through different roasting profiles to find the best flavour and aroma. We guarantee that if you tried the beans with different roasting profiles, they change so much that sometimes it can be quite difficult to choose which profile to run with. As the beans slowly rotate, the kernels lose moisture, which creates steam and loosens them from the husks.

03 Cracking and organizing Once the roasted beans have cooled down, we separate the husks and nibs by passing them through the Crankandstein, a tool which has three steel rolls where the beans get cracked. They then channel down to the big sieves below, which allow us to organize the pieces into four different sizes to make the next step more efficient.

04 Winnowing As husks are lighter than nibs, we use the power of wind and gravity to separate them. We turn on the vacuum that is connected to the winnower and nibs fall down the first tube, and husks down the second tube.

05 Pre-grind milling Even though our production is micro-scale, the amount of nibs is quite tough for our small, two-litre stone grinder. We need to mill the nibs into a paste before refining them.

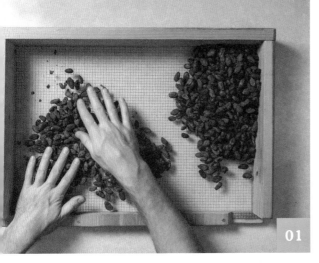

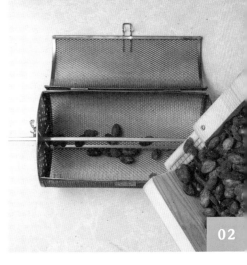

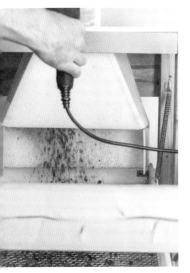

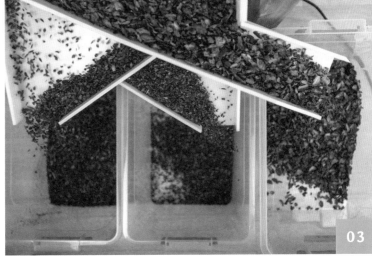

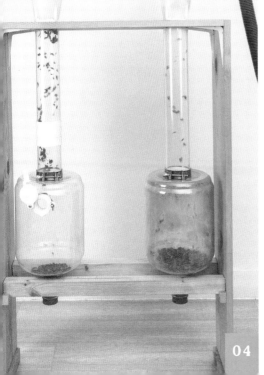

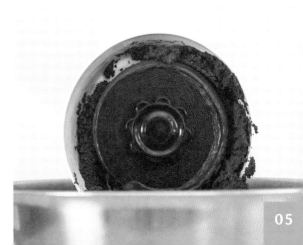

06 The twelve-hour grind For smooth, rich, and unctuous chocolate we need to grind the nib paste smaller than what your tongue can feel, which is twenty-five microns (0.025 mm). The grinding machine, also known as the wet grinder or 'melangeur', consists of two wheels spinning on top of a stone base. Wheels spin and the particle sizes reduce. Friction heats the resulting cocoa butter and turns it into cocoa liquor. After twelve hours of grinding, the liquor becomes fluid, and at this point we add two ingredients: sugar and a little bit of cocoa butter, which help achieve the texture we want.

07 Conching This is the fine-tuning of the chocolate process, the last step where we can alter the flavour and the viscosity of the chocolate. We simply release the pressure of the stone wheels to create heat and movement. The chocolate is aerated and unwanted volatile components, acidity, and astringency removed. We have to be careful at this stage that we don't conch too much, as this can reduce those fine flavours from Malaysia.

08 Tempering To us, a good chocolate bar is all about the sharp snap, beautiful shine, smooth texture, and taste. This is why tempering is important. Tempering is playing with temperatures. If chocolate isn't tempered properly it will look dull, sugar will bloom on the surface, and it will crumble when you snap. First, we heat the chocolate high enough to melt the different types of cocoa butter crystals. This cools to form the type of cocoa butter crystals that we need to make the bar shiny and give it a great-sounding, sharp snap. Afterwards, we raise the temperature again to help those crystals to spread evenly through the chocolate.

09 Moulding Our signature chocolate bar transforms the tradition of chocolate into a modern, sensory encounter. We researched and tested different designs, shapes, and thicknesses to give you a new chocolate experience. At the centre of each chocolate bar is a cacao pod-inscribed tablet, a little branded 'prize' to work towards. It is shareable, fun to break, and at the same time it has an unusual shape that fits comfortably on the palate, melts evenly, and tingles your taste buds.

SINGLE ORIGIN

Single origin means simply that the beans come from one place. This can mean one plantation or, more commonly, one region or country. Each plantation contains unique flavour profiles depending on the climate, soil, topography, harvest, fermentation, and drying methods. These are all things we take massively into account to ensure we achieve the right flavour for our bars. It is worth noting that the term 'single origin' does not necessarily equate to high quality chocolate; the chocolate making process also has a huge impact, so if you want to make sure you are consuming a quality product you need to check the makers behind the bar as well.

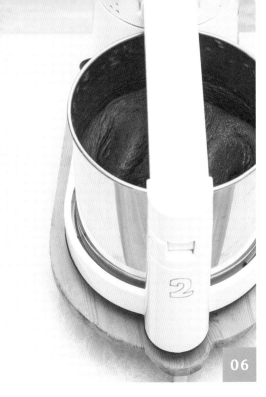

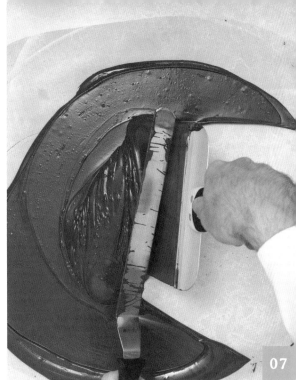

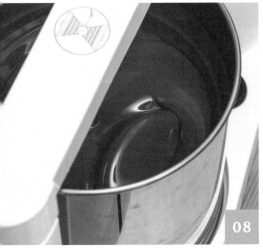

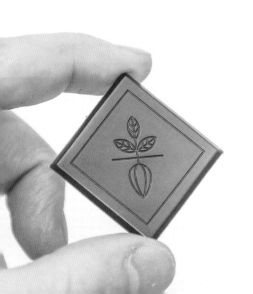

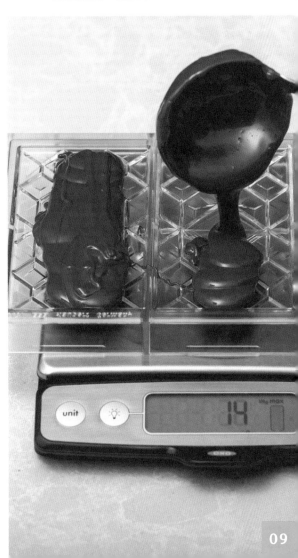

THE INTEGRITY OF DESIGN

Joy and happiness radiate with chocolate; it makes people happy, it paints smiles, it can mean the world to someone. And that moment when it does, we know we have done something right.

At the same time, tastes are subjective and diverse across the globe; each one of us has our own concept of what tastes good, what looks good, what's right from wrong. Our chocolate is made from hand-picked cocoa beans with no additional flavourings, but the origin of our beans does mean that they produce those delicious 'spicy' notes you may find in some chocolates. We make chocolate with curiosity, and we want people to be curious about our chocolate. Conserving the unique characteristic of the bean is a priority, which is why we choose to make only single-origin chocolate.

The creative process is a large part of making it all happen. We were not happy with regular bars of chocolate; we wanted to create something with meaning, so we brainstormed what we didn't like about generic chocolate bars and how we could maximize and improve upon this. We handed over a brief to our friend Adam Gill, who is a talented 3D designer we also met in New Zealand. As chocolate is a very malleable product after melting and tempering it, it can take any shape and still have a shiny surface. It is a real opportunity to create something unique and beautiful. However, the tricky part was getting the right shape and thickness to melt evenly in your mouth, and ensuring a sharp snap that is like music to your ears. We were given a remarkable design beyond our expectations.

We felt the same way about our packaging: how could we integrate it into our brand and ethos? Both our chocolate bar design and packaging are influenced by our travels finding cocoa farmers in Malaysia. Each wrapper features patterns influenced by textiles from Borneo and colour palettes inspired by the bars' tasting notes, all printed on beautifully foiled, recycled paper. We want our chocolate to proudly carry the culture of where it comes from.

However, packaging is an ongoing issue with confectionary products. You can see and find all sorts of methods executed and we wanted to avoid wasteful, non-enjoyable experiences. It is the first thing people see, and we wanted the consumer to feel special. We wanted it to stimulate each of those senses: first the eyes, then touch, smell, sound, and taste. Alongside this, we had to make conscious choices in materials and methods that considered today's global problems like waste and climate change. We are therefore looking to make it one hundred per cent compostable. We do not want to participate in catastrophic pollution generated by packaging, and it is a very nice idea to think that after people make our chocolate disappear the packaging will also disappear into a compost pile, which might even be use to grow cacao trees. We want to close the loop.

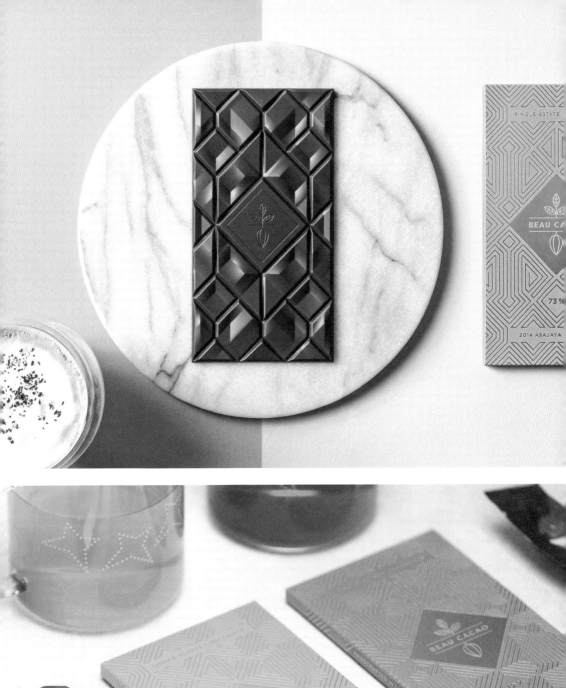

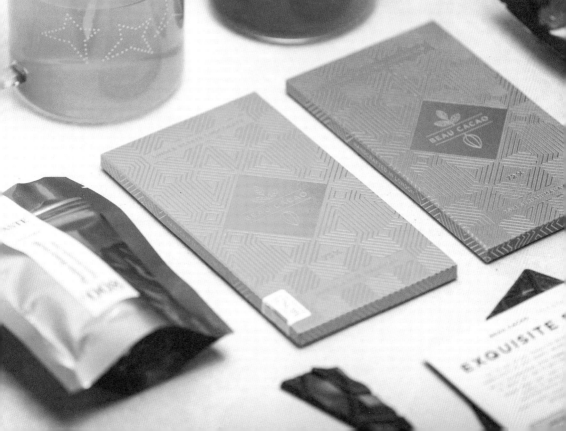

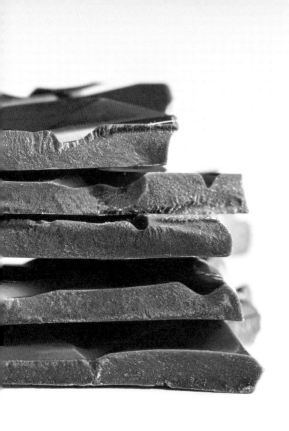

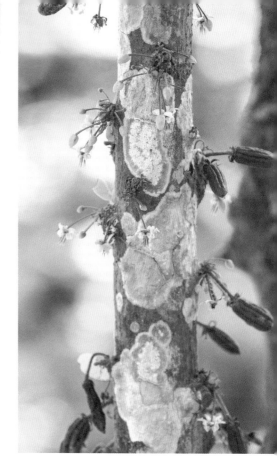

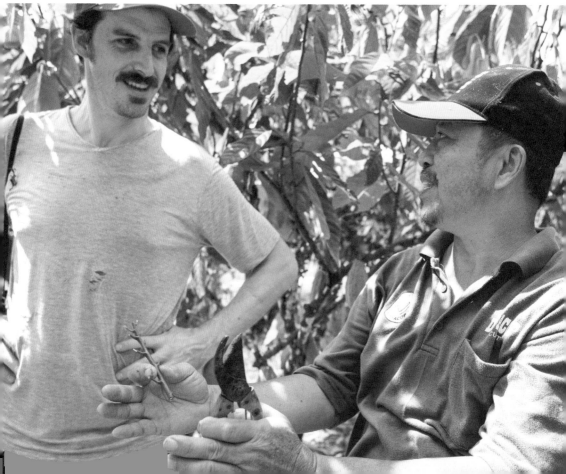

STARTING SMALL, THINKING BIG

The very first time we made chocolate was during our studies. We carried out multiple tests with some random cocoa beans (which in 2013 were quite difficult to find) and shared the chocolate with our friends, family, and colleagues; it all started from there. People were curious and that inspired us to pursue our newly found craft. This was just the start of our new beginning.

Making a living from chocolate when you want to control the whole process from farmer to consumer is not quite as easy as it looks or sounds. Sourcing and finding the ingredients ourselves and buying or making the machines necessary to make chocolate is very expensive. We wanted to ensure the product stood out from what was already available on the market, so we invested a lot of time and money in the design process. We both decided that one of us should stop working and dedicate ourselves to the craft, while the other continued working in their profession. This helps us support ourselves, and gives us the chance to create the brand and chocolate bar we dreamed of.

Selling directly to customers online worldwide has been our main strategy to date, with a handful of retailers. For now it is small, but it is a great way for us to learn without stress, and enables us to interact and engage with customers.

> "People were curious and that inspired
> us to pursue our newly found craft"

As mentioned above, if you want to start your own craft food business, there can be a lot of initial outlay in terms of equipment. Once we were happy with our chocolate design, we needed to find a polycarbonate mould supplier to create the moulds we would use. These don't come off the shelf, so we had to take time to research and ask other people and companies for recommendations. Creating a minimum viable chocolate product at a micro-scale means it is challenging to find efficient machines that fit in a home-scale business. Choices are limited, and we have had to improvise, make, and modify most of our tools. For example, our two-litre *melangeur* is mainly used for Indian specialities and is not supposed to run for forty-eight to seventy-two hours non-stop, so we had to modify it to handle chocolate. Another example is making new machines from scratch. Winnowers are expensive, but they are an integral part of the micro-scale process that need to be extremely efficient in separating the husks from the nibs cleanly and produce less waste. We looked at different technologies and created our own, which saved us a significant amount of money.

We are still using these modified machines and tools today. They make us understand more about each step of the process, help us grow as people, and cost a fraction of the price. Knowing the key components of making your craft is vital and is central to making informative decisions when your craft starts to scale up.

UPSCALING

Upscaling a craft is an interesting topic because there is a hard line between what we say is crafted and what is industrialized. We would like to think craft means someone has a special skill set and is attentive to every detail, big and small. If one is industrialized, it is debatable whether it still comes under the craft category, as each of those small details we care about could be lost along the process. Moving from traditional methods of production to fully automated machinery can in some cases ameliorate the texture and flavour. However, there are really big benefits to technological innovation: it can help to build a sustainable business by improving production efficiency and lessening labour intensity, while facilitating the reduction of our impact in our evolving world where we need to adapt. Ultimately, you have to weigh up the quality, environmental impact, and commercial viability and decide what feels right to you.

> "Knowing the key components of making your craft is vital and is central to making informative decisions"

LEGISLATION CHALLENGES

Legislation can often be time-consuming, and we would recommend contacting your local health and safety department right from the start. Our first legislation challenge was actually the packaging; the rules are not written clearly and depending on the size of your business, rules can change. It is important to make sure you are well informed, because reprinting packaging in large batches can be a costly mistake.

Exporting and importing your own ingredients is also an interesting challenge. The very first time we imported cocoa beans from Malaysia it took us two weeks to organize, and that wasn't the end of the story! We were the first private cocoa buyers that the Malaysian Cocoa Board had to deal with, and the export process was a little unknown for everyone. We met different people from different organizations for exporting rules. If we had to give one piece of advice for this kind of thing, it would be that you should get an appointment with the most senior person that you can. Even with exporting goods, find yourself a reliable and recommended freight agent that lays out each cost so you don't have an expensive surprise at the end.

TEAMWORK

We come from very different backgrounds and have very different skill sets that naturally came together when creating our chocolate brand. It is definitely a huge learning curve and we always make decisions collectively. For example, one of us makes chocolate throughout the day and when the other one comes back from work, we sit down, taste the results, and iterate the recipes to reach the desired flavour profile. When one is working on the design, we discuss the direction it is going in and commit to an idea. Communication is extremely important in building a newly found career.

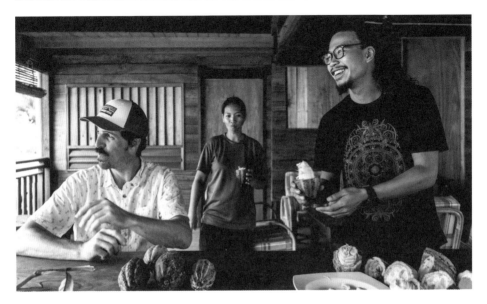

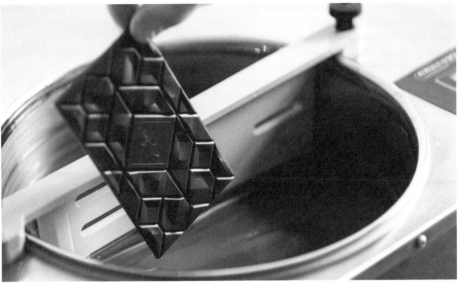

CONNECTING

The movement surrounding craft chocolate is a great community that allows us to feel grounded and connected, not only to what we eat, but to the people we share it with – customers or loved ones. It is certainly a magic ingredient that binds us together. It is important to keep this craft alive and share our invaluable knowledge in order to not lose the happiness we have gained from the craft chocolate movement.

We wouldn't be where we are today without this movement. There are affordable courses, great books, and online forums to learn from. People are keen to ask questions, share their experience, and now chocolate makers are even giving workshops. We are encouraged to educate others about how we make our chocolate by being transparent about every step through our website and social media channels.

> "Opening a chocolate bar is like opening a book. Looking beyond that next chocolate bar you eat will guarantee you an exciting story filled with a real adventure across the globe"

Social media is a great tool to give you a voice among the big brands. It is truly invaluable and helps us reach a high number of potential customers. Our effort online resulted in orders around the world just one month after launching. It was a real reward after working on our idea for three years! If we had to communicate using traditional, mainstream advertising methods, this would be near impossible, and wouldn't even be covered by our budget. Thanks to these modern tools, we are able to share our stories and get Beau Cacao recognized and grow our following globally, making us feel connected to an audience that is particularly interested in crafted products. As we work alone, it always helps to know that what we do is appreciated, and it keeps our motivation up and running during those difficult days we may encounter.

We are always aiming high to adhere to our core brand values, and we cater to the audience with our real stories from each product because people want transparency, to feel good, and to be guilt free. Making a product with meaning will naturally attract the right type of audience. Opening a chocolate bar is like opening a book. Looking beyond that next chocolate bar you eat will guarantee you an exciting story filled with a real adventure across the globe, and you can be connected to many people from very different backgrounds who all share a common goal and have a strong relationship with our Earth.

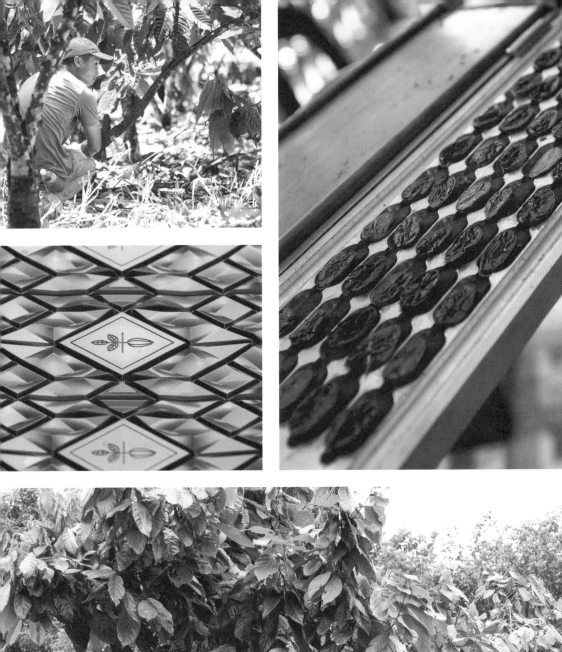
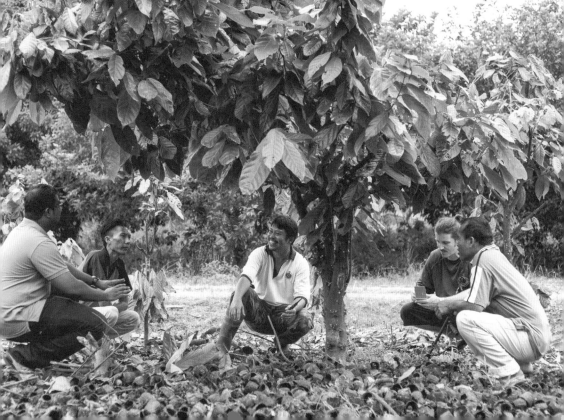

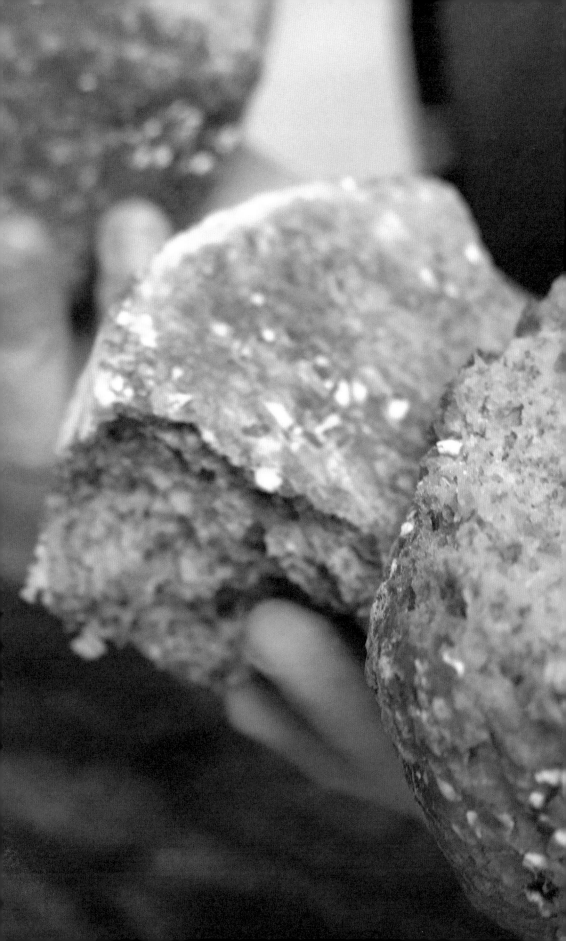

BREAD

Bread is one of our oldest foods. Traditionally, it was a wholesome and simple food, often made by hand at home. The 1960s drastically changed all this with the invention of the Chorleywood bread process in Britain. Bread became a cheap, mass-produced commodity. The once-natural process was transformed almost beyond recognition by the addition of chemical enzymes and additives, and sped up by high-speed mechanical mixers, resulting in a spongy and low-cost product that can withstand days on the supermarket shelf.

Artisan bread is the proper stuff: nourishing, comforting, and made by hand often using only flour, water, salt, and yeast as a base. It has been allowed the time it needs to ferment, for the natural enzymes to react slowly with the flour. The result is a healthier bread with a rich texture that is enjoyable to eat and kinder to our bodies.

"Historically, bread in one of its many forms has been central to many people's lives worldwide, whether that be of religious, cultural, or nutritional value"

Alan Davis, The Authentic Bread Company

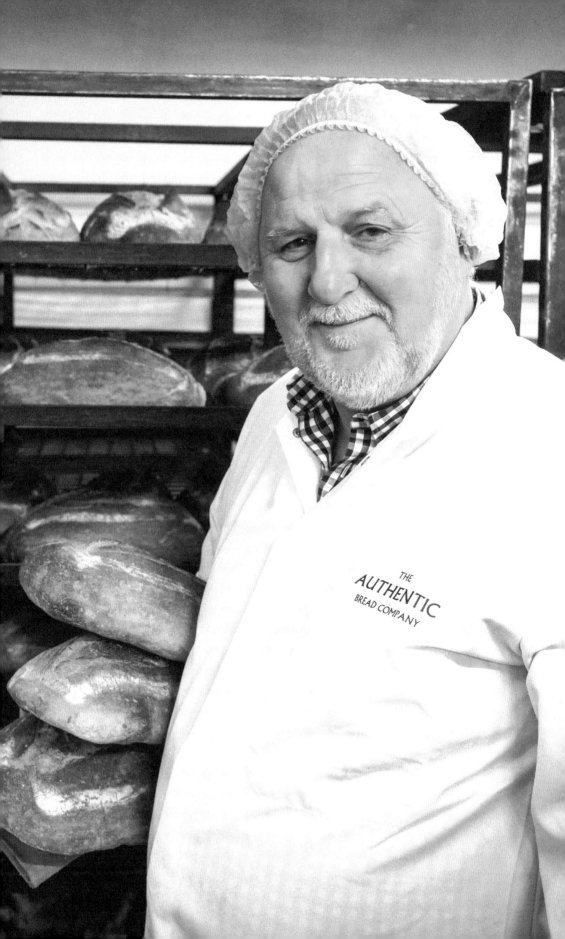

THE AUTHENTIC BREAD COMPANY

ALAN DAVIS

Newent, Gloucestershire | authenticbread.co.uk

My original career as a BT Engineer was a long way from craft baking. My wife and I were lucky enough to take our children on family holidays to France where we all enjoyed the bread so much more than at home and the cultural approach to baking was so far removed from the mass-produced, joyless bread generally available at that time in the UK.

A family friend managed a flour mill, and encouraged my interest in making bread in the traditional way – that is, using basic ingredients and leaving the bread doughs to ferment without the use of flour treatment agents. As soon as we had made our first loaves I was hooked. Being able to make such wonderful produce from four simple ingredients was inspiring and led me to try new techniques and flavours. When I was offered the chance of redundancy from BT in 1995 after more than twenty-five years, it seemed like a natural progression to turn my real passion for craft baking from hobby to profession, so I converted my double garage into a small bakery.

It was a terrifying prospect, with four children and a mortgage, but the confidence I had in our products drove me onwards. After winning the top organic award from the Soil Association for our olive bread in our first year, the business went from strength to strength. We now bake a variety of breads, cakes, and pastries. All our products are vegetarian and, with the exception of some of our cakes and pasties, most are vegan too.

THE IMPORTANCE OF PROVENANCE

We believe passionately that provenance and quality of food are key to health and well-being. Mass-produced bread typically has a list of around fourteen ingredients, whereas our basic recipe made by hand has around four. It is time consuming, and the work is physically demanding, but the resulting quality of the bread shows the care and attention that is lavished on it.

We use only organic ingredients in our bread, and the certification of an ingredient as organic is only made if there are the necessary quality and ethical assurances. Organic, as we see it, is the assurance of good quality and good methodology. With news in 2018 concerning glyphosates (weedkiller) being found in bread products, we know we are vindicated in our commitment to the organic philosophy. Organic promotes a healthy environment as well as great animal welfare, as do we.

As a BRC (British Retail Consortium)-accredited organization, we have an additional responsibility to know where our ingredients originate, and how they are produced. We must trace all of our ingredients back to their original producers, and require information on how they are produced. We keep as much as we can local and therefore in plain sight, but the nature of our business demands that much of what we use is imported. For example, wheat grown in Britain may not have the necessary protein content to make bread reliably when used alone. We don't use any artificial agents in our bread and therefore we need to ensure that the protein content is as high as possible to produce good bread. Additionally, we are limited in Britain for organically grown wheat and therefore what we use comes from Europe in the main, although we purchase the flour itself from local millers. We produce over 300 different products, and obviously to service this variety we need many different ingredients, again with organic certification. We therefore often need to cast our net a little further to ensure we can bring fresh and innovative products to our customers. Our methods of tracking back to source can give us the information we need on the sustainability and ethical production of our ingredients. That said, there are also a lot of ingredients that we do source locally, such as butter, eggs, and nearly two tonnes of Herefordshire apples each year.

As our business has grown over the last twenty-five years, we have seen an unprecedented increase in the number of customers who want to understand the provenance of their food, and the producers behind it. This has been both reassuring and exciting for us, to share our passion with our customers, and extol the benefits of making bread the old-fashioned way. Working in the organic industry in particular has brought us together with like-minded food producers. We have a great community of people around us who are passionate about how we fuel ourselves. Organic and good quality really are synonymous, and as the organic movement goes from strength to strength and the market expands, we see many new and exciting ingredients available organically, which allows us to create more innovative products.

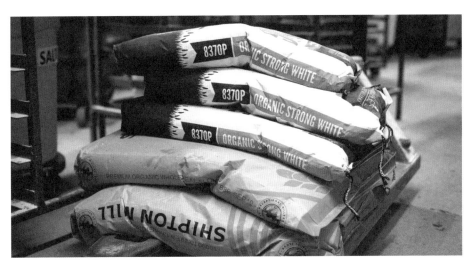

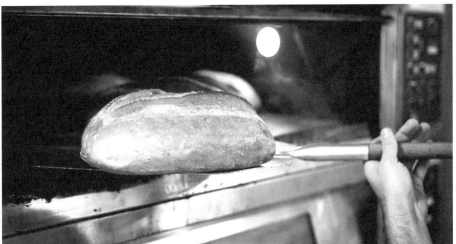

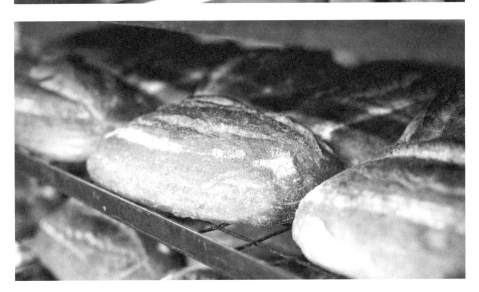

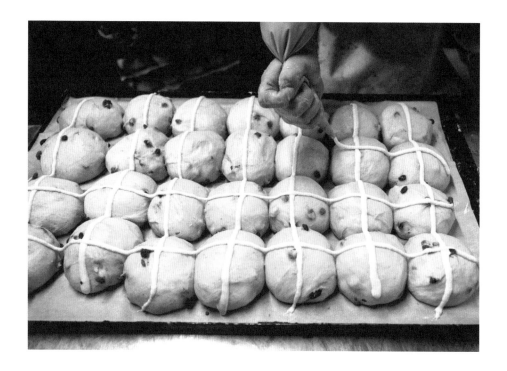

BREAD AS A BUSINESS

From working alone in my garage at night and my wife Jane making the deliveries, to our current team of twenty-five, we have always held the belief that it was possible to make a reasonable living from baking. It hasn't always been a lot and it certainly hasn't always been easy, but as three of my four children now manage the day-to-day running of the business – which is marvellous for me to see – I can feel proud that there is a legacy that will go on supporting their families too.

Unfortunately, bread has been so badly devalued by both the mass-produced methods of production, and by the price wars of the supermarkets, that making a good living in this industry is undeniably tough. We are very conscious of keeping our costs reasonable, but this does have to be balanced with rewarding and retaining our skilled employees. As so much is performed by hand, our labour costs are enormous compared with, say, a plant bakery, but most importantly this shines through in the quality of the end product.

When I first started this business, I envisioned a simple life as a local country baker; little did I expect that it would grow to the extent it has. As it has grown, so has the workload and considerations for labelling, ingredients, and many other details that people possibly don't immediately think of when they first set up an enterprise.

With our current commitments we are generally busy throughout the year, but have some slightly quieter periods. However, around sixty per cent of our business is now compressed into the three-month Christmas period. It is a fundamental part of our business as Christmas is a time that a lot of people really treat themselves to the finest produce, hence the huge uplift in our production. Last year we made over 800,000 mince pies entirely by hand, which is obviously incredibly hard work!

There are two main parts to the company: there are the core local shops that we deliver to and the large online retailers who distribute our products all over the country. The latter is now the larger portion of the business, and is a vital way of making sure that we can reach as many customers as possible. Sadly the days of artisan bread being widely available on many local high streets are largely gone, but working with distributors allows us to provide customers with a viable alternative.

Often the assumption is that having your own business is a dream of flexibility that gives ultimate power over one's own destiny. It does to a greater extent, but with such flexibility comes enormous commitment – the buck ultimately stops with you. I would absolutely encourage everyone to follow their dreams, but with a cautionary tale of the strain that such a commitment can put on you, and those around you. You will have to make great sacrifices, and take great risks, but the ultimate reward can be a flourishing business that represents your dedication to your beliefs and processes.

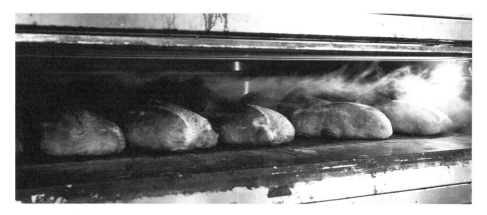

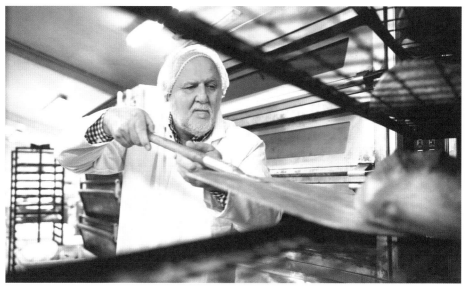

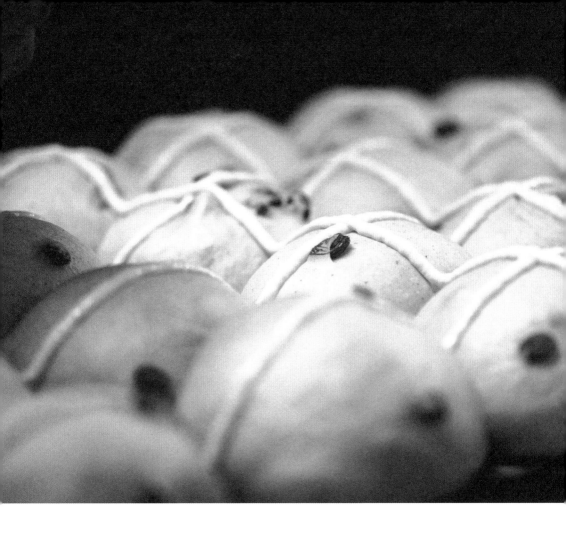

SURVIVING IN THE MODERN WORLD

It must be pointed out then that cost is a limiting factor for any producer – there is no limit to a craftsman's creativity but it cannot be at any cost to our customers. That said, we have, over the years, made sure that we consider the ultimate cost when developing our products so that there are no late surprises, or wasted costs when a more expensive product goes to market. We would love to spend all of our time creating in a test kitchen, but ultimately our financial and operational resources must be well spent in ensuring a sustainable business. As we are a small team leading the business we have to be mindful of our priorities. We now have to produce within cost boundaries, and within the legislative requirements that sometimes can curb creativity, but we stand reassured that we lay good foundations which work efficiently and can allow us to develop and grow in the way that we need to.

Our business is fairly niche, in that we are producing in volume without compromising on our commitment to traditional methods. This demands a little exceptional thinking, and some flexible approaches to scheduling our manufacture, but with the support of our team we do achieve it. We have had to adapt some methods in order to achieve our volume supply – mainly relating to scheduling and time management – but crucially this will never be at the expense of our quality. We still use minimal machinery because we believe that a loaf untouched by human hands is a joyless thing.

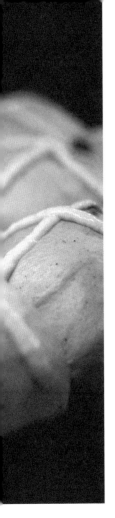
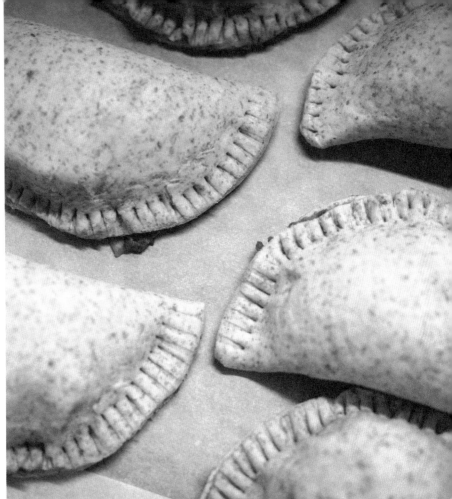

Additionally, mechanizing the process would mean we would have to compromise on the composition and ingredients in order to take any variability out of the process, which simply goes against our core values. Innovation to accommodate high-volume manufacture is always welcome in our organization, but we truly believe that this can be achieved – albeit with very significant effort – without resorting solely to mechanization.

When production levels begin to compromise quality of the end product or our approach to sourcing and staffing our organization, that will be the point at which we draw back. As long as we continue to make great products, made from great ingredients, and nurture and support our employees, we are where we should be.

"We believe that a loaf untouched by human hands is a joyless thing"

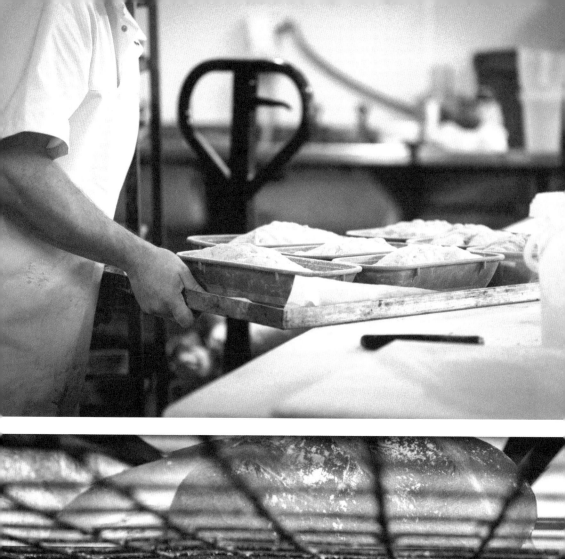
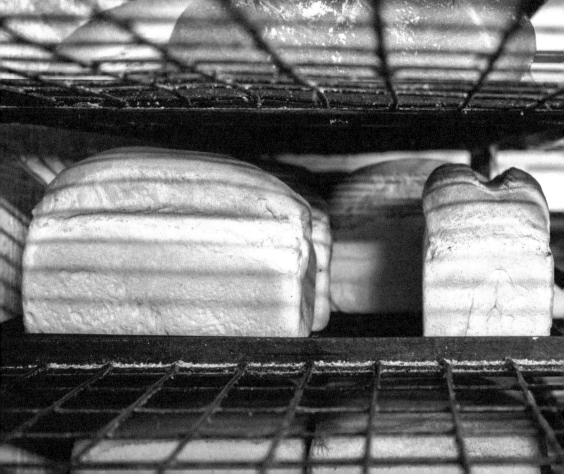

HOW OUR BREAD IS MADE

The secret ingredient in the perfect loaf is time. Our time-honoured traditional methods allow the doughs to develop slowly and let the yeasts produce flavour that gives our breads their unique character. Although the process is long, the difference between this and Chorleywood processed breads – where artificial improvers are used to speed up the process – is remarkable.

Our breads begin with their mother, our starter Miranda, which is around nineteen years old now. We mix our starter into a leaven, which then develops over twenty-four hours. The starter is just a mix of flour and water, where bacteria and yeasts are encouraged to develop. A leaven is a mix of flour and the starter which causes the bread to rise in the absence of other yeasts

The leaven is then combined with the simple ingredients of flour, water, and salt. The dough is mixed over a period of time to encourage water absorption and to develop the gluten.

We then allow the dough to ferment for around three hours to develop the flavour. While it is in fermentation, we gently fold the dough to stretch the gluten and encourage the yeast to start working.

The dough is then left to rise. This part of the process is known as proving, where the bread is placed in a warm damp atmosphere to allow the yeast to convert sugar, gluten, and protein in the flour to CO_2 and alcohol, producing bubbles that form the textured crumb of a loaf and allow it to rise.

The loaves are then hand-moulded to retain the air and texture. This process is lengthy and sticky with the wet dough, but eventually the loaves are shaped and then make their way to the proofing baskets.

Once proved, we bake our loaves in our wood-fired ovens to give a crisp crust.

FOOD SAFETY

The Authentic Bread Company has a BRC A grade accreditation – one of only a handful of businesses of our size to reach such a standard. Commitment to food safety is a central and critical part of our business and we believe that this attitude should be shared by all food producers, whether they look to such formal approval or not. For example, we ensure staff all wear protective personal equipment, follow hygiene regulations, and carry out contamination control practices. We don't use any high-risk ingredients (such as meat), but traceability and allergen control are central to considering the safety of our customers. Along with our certification by the Soil Association, the workload and therefore the cost of making the commitment to food safety is huge, but one that we feel is ultimately worthwhile. Being a risk to public health has no place in any organization, regardless of its size, but often a small business can feel the burden of such costs, which are largely hidden from the consumer. Having recently visited a bakery where these risks were being taken, our investment in pest control, traceability, and foreign body control (to name a few) was reaffirmed.

It is very important in our business to keep abreast of changes in legislation for labelling and food safety. Food labelling is an area of significant media interest, and it is essential that we comply fully with the legal requirements to clearly disclose ingredients, particularly those that can affect allergies. Again, the cost of labelling all of our products is enormous, and learning how to keep up to date with rapidly changing requirements such as nutritional analysis has become necessary. The frustration we have is when we see many other businesses failing to comply with regulations, but not suffering any consequences for doing so.

EMPLOYEE HEALTH & SAFETY

Health and safety are critical for all businesses – of course we must guarantee the safety of our staff, but with enormous and increasing legislation, becoming experts in this has been a challenging area of the business. Crucially, you are also working with human beings who, as rapid developers, seek the most streamlined approach to their work. It is therefore a challenge to ensure that the procedures are always followed in the safest way without demeaning people's skills and effort.

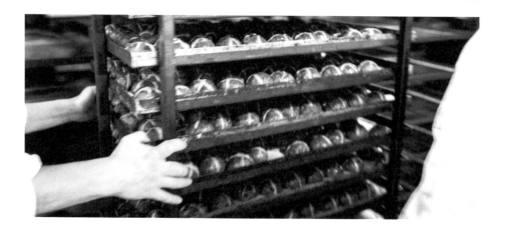

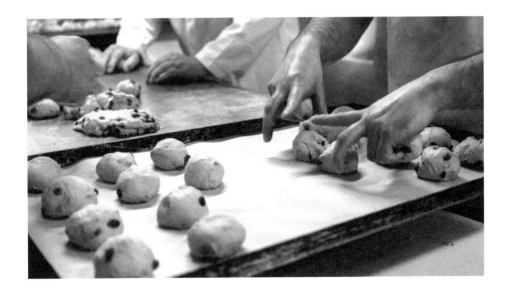

PACKAGING

We are always thinking about how to package our products, both to give the best possible bread life to the customer and also to do so in a sustainable way. Packaging our products ensures their organic credentials remain intact all the way to the consumer. This means that it prevents any contamination. For example, I once saw unwrapped organic bread at a market sitting in uncovered baskets. A car was parked up beside it with fumes being blown onto the bread, which brings its organic credentials into question.

We incorporate a range of eco-minded packaging – all of our packaging is recyclable and we use cardboard and paper products wherever possible. We have to balance this with our products reaching customers in the best possible condition, and ultimately we have to mitigate the staling of our goods. In addition we minimize packaging wherever we can. Internally we also participate fully in recycling services and minimize landfill with a 'manufacture to order policy'.

When David Attenborough reached our screens with *Blue Planet II* in 2017, we shared the horror of what was happening in our oceans because of plastics. We have, however, tried to make a considered approach rather than a knee-jerk reaction. Plastics play a very important role in the food industry, but in today's context we are looking to reduce our use of them. We looked at paper bags, but they took moisture from the product, so after much deliberation we are looking to move to a fully compostable material for packaging our bread. This comes from sustainable sources, and breaks down fully with no residues, so in theory is the best environmental solution. Even if the customer doesn't compost it at home, we have reassurance that it will break down quickly and completely. However, this technology will come at some financial cost, that being around four times as expensive as alternatives. We hope that our customers will see the value in this, and that the benefit outweighs the increased cost, but the ultimate impact remains to be seen.

THE VALUE OF CRAFT BAKERS

The baking industry has taken innumerable knocks since the invention of the Chorleywood bread process and no-time dough methods. Baking was dominated by improvers, preservatives, and pre-mixes, and the removal of any variable factors by applying these additions reduced the need for any kind of baking skill. The majority of loaves purchased in the UK have never been touched by human hands, processed instead between silos and travelling ovens, wrapped in plastic, and delivered to the supermarket shelves.

As this trend grew, so the number of baking jobs reduced, and of course this was soon followed by a reduction in the number of skilled bakers, and almost a total absence of new recruits coming into the industry. I was self-taught to a greater extent, but my passion and business ultimately were borne from a hobby and something that I enjoyed doing. There was little to bring new bakers into this career. Sourcing skilled bakers in the past has taken us to business-limiting situations – where we had the work and customers, but simply could not find skilled people. We have an excellent team now but we have fought hard to find them – many come from Eastern Europe, as the baking industry still thrives there. Therefore, passing on skills is utterly imperative to prevent us from only having mass-produced bread available.

As a smaller business, in a very cost-focused market, we struggle to compete with supermarkets and bigger brands. We have, however, reached the conclusion that we should not try to compete as such. We know our products are special, and that most mass-produced food pales into insignificance next to produce that is made with the best ingredients and total commitment to quality and traditional methods. Instead, we try to seek out like-minded people who value what we do and how we do it. The challenge is always getting our goods to all of those people, who may be few and far between. Our range of supply has never been larger than now, and with fantastic distributors who ultimately share our ethos we can reach more customers than ever before.

We hope that our products tell a story – that being our story. We would like to think that the customer will appreciate how we have developed our methods, business, people, and practices with a passion, hard work, and a commitment to our beliefs. We truly believe that our products stand apart and while the route to get here has been long, hard, and has often sent ripples through our family life, we have all worked hard to get here.

Bread – the 'staff of life' – has been our single most important staple for centuries, dating back in Britain to the coarse flatcakes of our prehistoric ancestors. The word 'lord' derives from the old English 'hlāford', meaning the keeper of bread. Historically, bread in one of its many forms has been central to many people's lives worldwide, whether that be of religious, cultural, or nutritional value. Like coffee it can be ubiquitous, featuring daily in many people's lives, whether it is chapati, baguette, pretzel, or lavash. Craft bakers like us keep this tradition alive against the tide of mass-produced bread now out there.

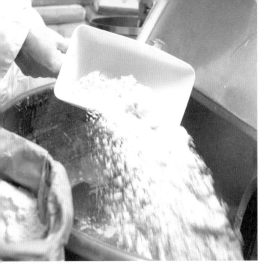
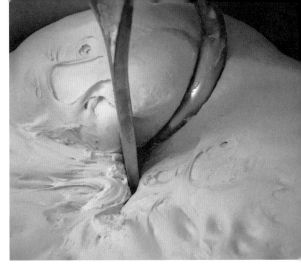
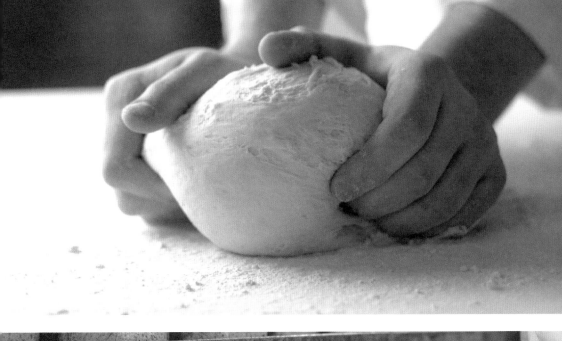
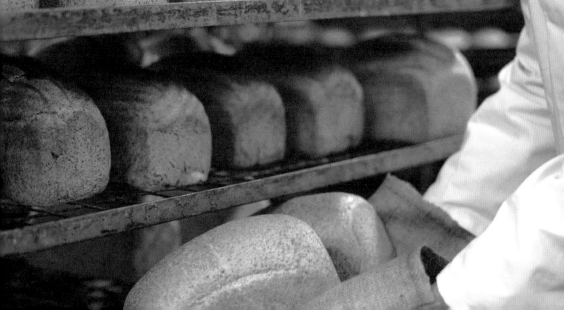

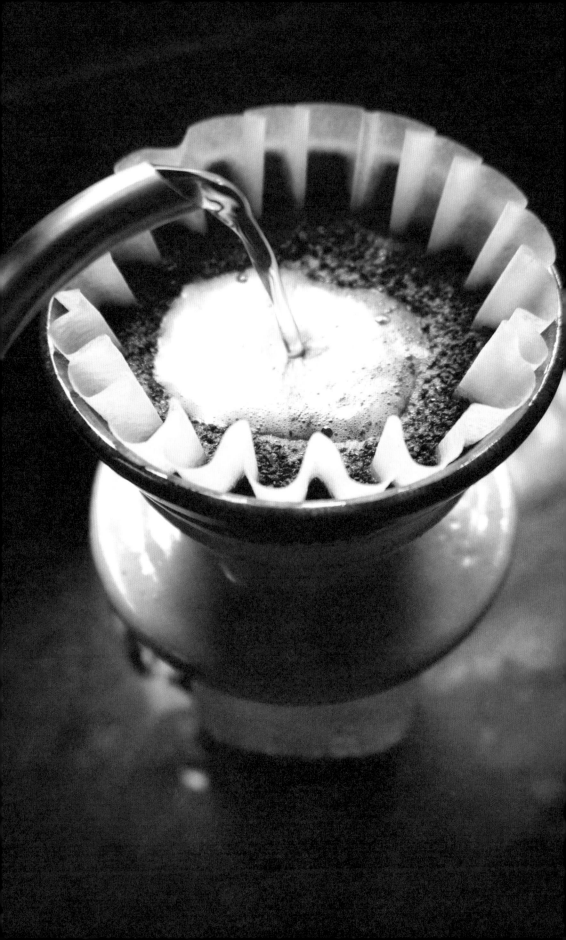

COFFEE

Coffee is all about the story, not least because the discovery of coffee is steeped in legend, with myth leading us to believe it was made by an Ethiopian goat-herder, Kaldi, who around 850 AD noticed that his goats became excitable after eating berries from a coffee plant. There is no way of verifying this, but coffee as a drink has certainly been circulating the globe since the fifteenth century at least.

What is really interesting about coffee is that because it is so process-driven, it compels a story to be told. Coffee is a craft from beginning to end, from the ripeness at which you choose to harvest the bean, to the way you decide to produce it. You can ferment it in different ways – with or without yeast; the way you roast it then dramatically changes the coffee again; then there is brewing it. This is why coffee is so complicated. There can be a craftsperson controlling it at each stage.

"Coffee is almost ubiquitous. It is incredible for us to be able to travel basically anywhere in the world and be able to talk with another fellow coffee person and feel a sense of kinship"

Brandon Damitz & Kelleigh Stewart, Big Island Coffee Roasters

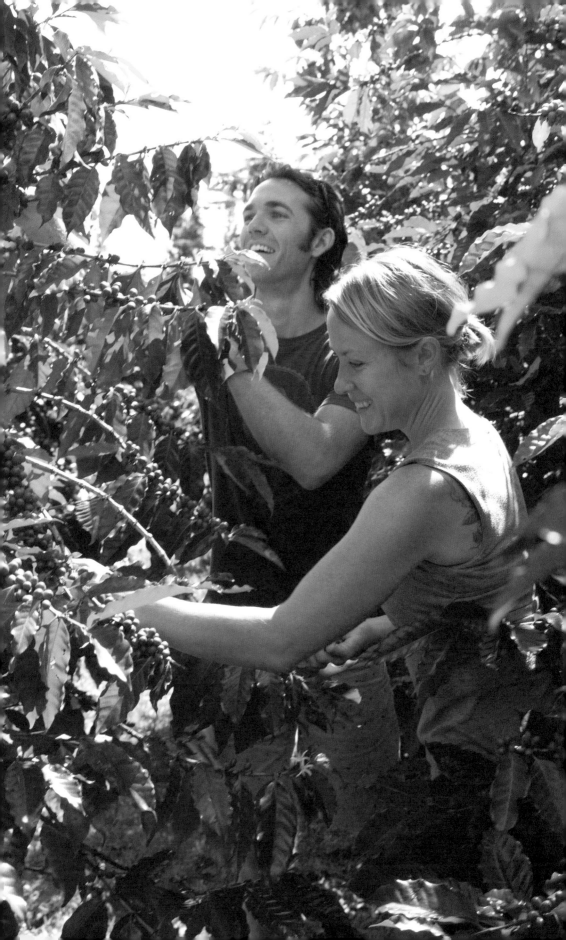

BIG ISLAND
COFFEE ROASTERS

BRANDON DAMITZ & KELLEIGH STEWART

Puna, Hawaii | bigislandcoffeeroasters.com

Our coffee is grown over a bed of lava that was laid down around 500 years ago. There is only about a foot of broken-up lava rock called cinder and then there is the coffee; we don't really have any soil or dirt – it is grown hydroponically with rainwater and fertilizer.[13]

Underneath all of our property is a huge lava tube. It is about forty miles long, like a cave. One day our friends were taking us through the lava tube and we spent about three hours down there, hiking from one area to another. There was a puddle of water dripping down from the ceiling, so we went over to drink it. We noticed that the water tasted a lot like our coffee did and realized it was because the roots of the coffee were embedded in the same matter that the water was filtering through. The roots were in the lava. That is our place and that is where we are, so we decided to name our coffee Puna Kazumura after the lava tube, the minerals of which help make the flavour in our coffee.

TRANSFORMATION AND GROWTH

Everyone has this one thing in common: we all want growth. We want either personal growth or family growth; we want to feel that there is progress or a positive change happening. When you are dealing with a raw product and you are refining it, you are changing it in a way that means it can be experienced in a new way, by a different community. That feels like progress, like learning and developing.

One of the best things about our craft is the engagement of the senses and using your body. Working with plants, being on the farm, roasting, cupping – it all keeps you active. You are just *being* in the pursuit of perfecting something by way of a process. And you are not only trying to perfect the process, you are trying to perfect yourself in that process too. This exchange is deeply gratifying and there is really no substitute for it. There is a humbling dance to be appreciated between trying something

> "One of the best things about our craft is the engagement of the senses and using your body"

and failing at it, and then learning, adjusting, and hopefully improving results with the next attempt. We are lucky in that we get to work in the whole process of coffee. We roast, we grow, we dry, we mill, we grade, we farm; it's the whole spectrum, the whole farm to cup in one spot. We both love immersing ourselves in something. It is empowering to have that sense of participation in the dynamics of a process like that. Working with your hands, carrying out iterative processes, and doing them over and over again, edges out any sort of anxiety that you might have; it can quiet any questions of purpose or meaning in your life. Everything feels in its place. Along with that satisfaction, which is deeply mentally, emotionally, psychologically, and spiritually satisfying, you can also feel in control of your own destiny a little bit – but also not (there is only so much you can do in the face of a hurricane!). It is unapologetic in so many respects, but it is also nurturing.

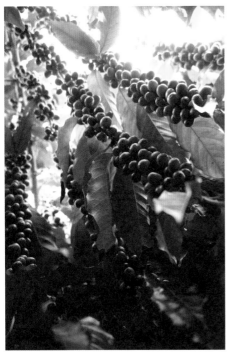
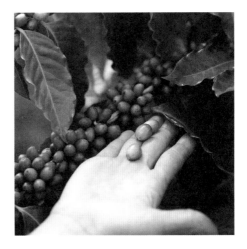
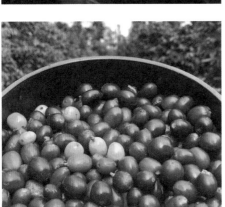
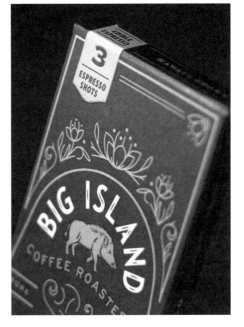
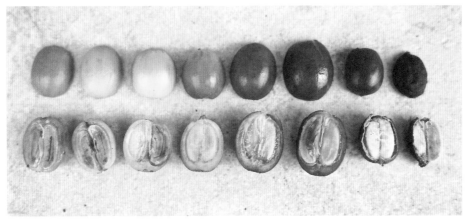

OUR BUSINESS

Part of our mission is to provide speciality-grade Hawaiian coffees, which means coffees that are of a premium quality. We have a high cost of living here, so Hawaiian coffees are likely to be more expensive than many others in the world. We therefore feel that we have a duty to make them higher quality and to source the best coffee because we don't have a choice about the price but we do have a choice about quality. We grow our own coffee but that is only a small portion of what we could potentially afford to grow; the coffees that we grow end up being our most boutique coffees – hand-harvested, hand-sorted, and only roasted once a month.

In addition to selling our own coffee, we also source coffees from around Hawaii. We try to connect those coffees with customers seeking something specific, so we like to think of ourselves as a connection between the customer and the farmer. We also work with farmers around Hawaii and roast their coffee in our style. We taste the coffee before we take it on to make sure it meets our specifications and then sell it. There are a lot of regions with different vintages in Hawaii and we want to showcase those regions. We also hold consultations with other producers and try to pass on what we have learned. Our income is therefore threefold.

OUR PLACE IN THE COMMUNITY

We have decided to work with other farmers in this way because it is fun and we enjoy this lifestyle. In Hawaii, being in such close proximity in a small community has meant that being involved in business is a delicate type of engagement, especially when we have friends who are direct competitors. The idea that we are going to be pitted against our neighbours, just so we can win, doesn't make sense to us, so we have been very open about sharing information and have become friends with many farmers. We are on the Hawaii Coffee Association Board of Directors, trying to help farmers improve their crop and communication with the public.

At the same time, what we love about crafting things and about having our own business is that it is an opportunity for self-expression. We are definitely promoters of collectives, but day-to-day the farming and the craft allows us to be who we are as people and amplify that in a way that nobody else can replicate. It is an illusion to think that we are all fighting against each other. That is more of a city-business concept, not a craftsperson-business concept.

One of the reasons we do business in Hawaii is to elevate the value of coffee here so that farmers can make a living. Coffee is such a social thing and is a big driver for community. As a topic, it can be highly cultural and personal, and not just from the perspective of the consumer; there is so much culture and personality associated with it at a farmer-to-farmer level too. Coffee is almost ubiquitous. It is incredible for us to be able to travel basically anywhere in the world and be able to talk with another fellow coffee person and feel a sense of kinship.

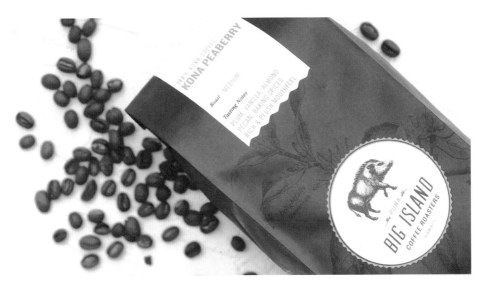

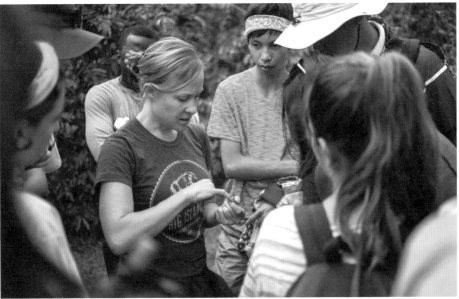

COFFEE AS CRAFT

With a craft you are injecting the product with who you are, so you are not really in competition with everyone you know. It is about style. We are not worried about someone trying to replicate our style because, frankly, we work really hard to make it tough to do that! If someone tried, I would just laugh and say good luck. But I would also counsel them and say you should do *you*; don't try to be somebody else. If you are not authentic with your process and you are not authentic with who you are, people will quickly spot you as bogus. The best advice is not to copy anyone else – just do your own thing. Be individualistic.

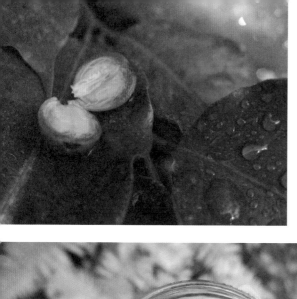
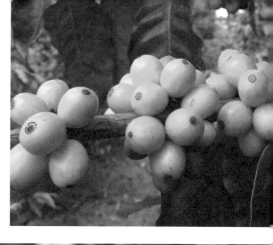
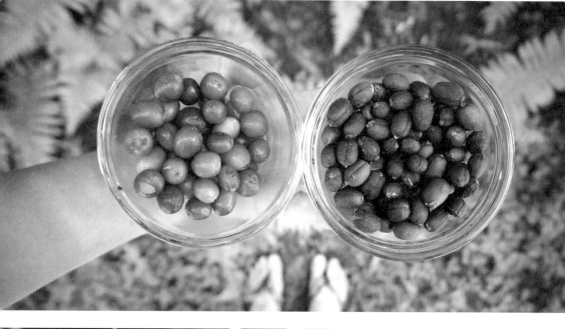
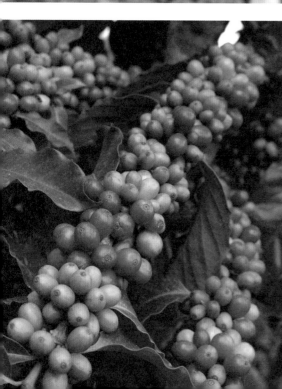
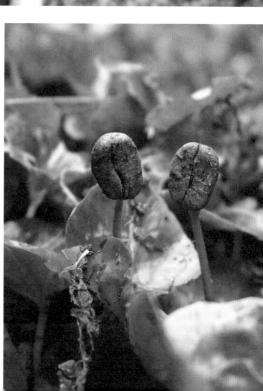

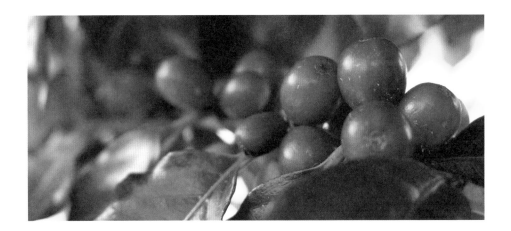

STARTING FROM SCRATCH

We started off not knowing anything about coffee or business. Brandon has a background in farming and when we both came across an overgrown coffee farm in Hawaii in 2010, we thought we would give it a go. We had the product and then had to work out how to sell it to people. So much of the process has been trial and error, learning as we go – it hasn't always been easy or fun. If we had our way we would be out with the coffee trees most of the time! But that is not the reality of it. Nine to five you are doing the thing you love, but after that you have to do all the things that come along with it. You have to keep things organized and afloat – you can end up feeling like a clown on a unicycle, on a tightrope, juggling! It is challenging but we are grateful for the process. Having to go from being solely a crafter to dealing with the business side of things is really a rite of passage for a craftsperson. You have to do it and there is no getting around it.

Before our business was growing and we were mainly outside harvesting coffee, we listened to podcasts and learned about business through these. We learned about health codes, legal issues, branding, packaging – we called it coffee college! It was like a four-year university course. As a result we can now make quick decisions because we have had the time to listen to people who are smarter than us, and to learn and research online.

THE POWER OF DESIGN

You can really learn to love things like marketing, branding, and design. In many ways, design that communicates your intention and your style in visuals is the most important thing a producer can do if they have a packaged good because people don't take the time to read labels. You have one second to pop off the shelf otherwise you are going to drown. This is something we have invested in that has returned on investment over and over again. Invest in great artists who can communicate who you are in great visuals.

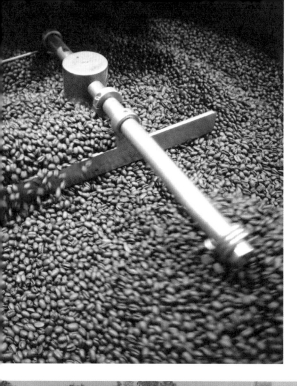

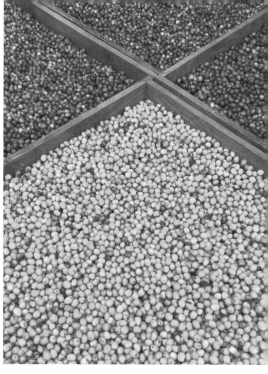

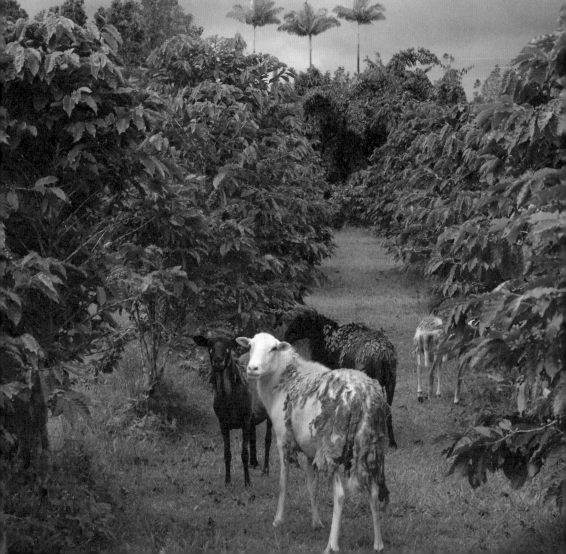

THE PRICE OF AGRICULTURE

Stepping away from the business administration element for a moment, it is important to point out that farming is far more demanding than people realize. It is also difficult to communicate to people how fragile the circumstances of this sort of business are and how much you can lose, even when you have worked so hard. You have no hope of controlling certain factors at all. For instance, a hurricane came through a few years ago and unfortunately hurricane season and harvest season overlapped. We had a lot of ripe coffee on the trees and then we had torrential rain – the coffee was washed off the trees, rotted away, and we lost about thirty per cent of our crop in a week. It was incredibly devastating.

Natural disaster is only one piece of the puzzle: you also have price fluctuations of inputs and the simple truth of demanding physical labour. It is frustrating to hear people complain about the price of agricultural goods, even in their most raw state.

In the romanticization of farming there is this beautiful gloss over what farmers do. As a result, you come across people who decide they want to go into farming and end up causing damage. For example, someone buys a cheap acre of land and bulldozes native trees to plant coffee. They find out a few years later how hard it is to grow coffee and they abandon the crop. You then get invasive species growing in its place. A couple of times a month we get emails saying: 'We just bought land in your area and want to grow coffee, what should we do?' We say: 'Don't do it!' – not because we want to discourage people from growing things, but because you need to organize the backend first. It's not all fairy tales and cupcakes: the market is saturated, and the price is high. It is no longer good enough to be revolutionary. You need to be a business person to make it work.

SUSTAINING YOURSELF

You need to sustain yourself to be able to sustain your practice – this is difficult to do when you are busy and there is not enough time. Self-care is important but it can be tricky to build this into your time. You can't say no to your agricultural crop. You don't know when there are going to be hurricanes, volcanoes, or leaks, so you are always on the go! This type of lifestyle is only for a certain type of person; you can't be lazy with this career.

If you can think of affordable ways to save time these are often worth doing. As an example, it is usually extra busy during the Christmas holiday season, as this is the time everyone wants their coffee and September/October to January/February also happens to be the coffee harvesting season. For this reason, we have now hired a chef to make our food so that we have enough time to eat over the holiday season.

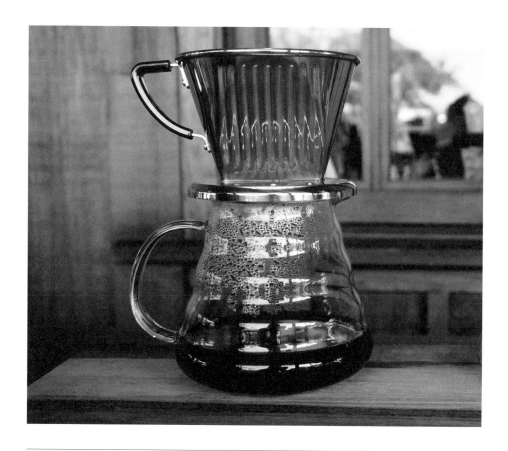

BROADENING MARKETS

There are two farmers' markets in our area. We used to sell at these but we do that less now, in the interest of time. Because the coffee is relatively expensive, most local people can't afford it, so we were relying on tourists coming in and buying it. With the natural disasters recently, however, fewer people have been visiting. Social media has helped with online sales since then and we have started to go to more food and trade shows – these are targeted shows with more foot traffic. It is good that we don't need to depend on farmers' markets. They are a great avenue for interaction, for people to get to know the farmers, and for farmers to get to know people. At the same time, it has definitely been a huge lifesaver and timesaver to be able to reach people outside Hawaii via e-commerce.

We wrote a business plan on the idea of moving beyond local sales because we have seen how focusing on one route of income can devastate business owners. We are in contact with other farmers about how to work with technology. You basically have two choices with technology: you can ignore it or embrace it. We have found that technology – particularly in the form of e-commerce – has allowed us to live the way we want to live. It enables us to distribute outside Hawaii, because if we depend on tourists and they stop coming then we can't feed ourselves. If there is a natural disaster and you just focus on farmers' markets then you are not going to survive.

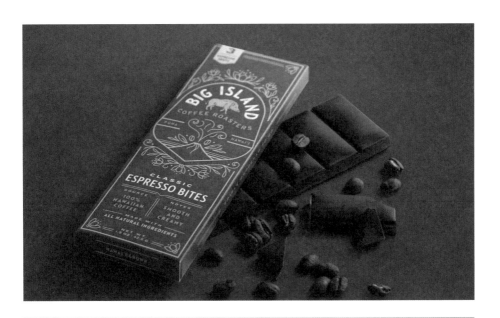

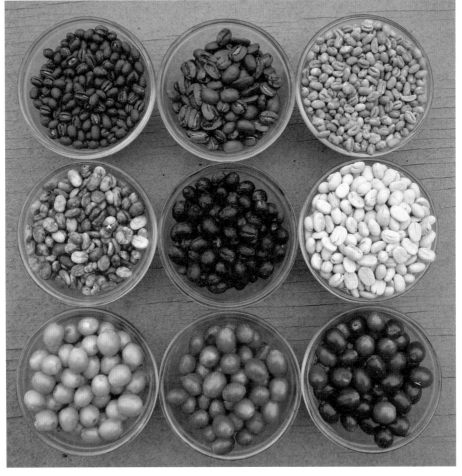

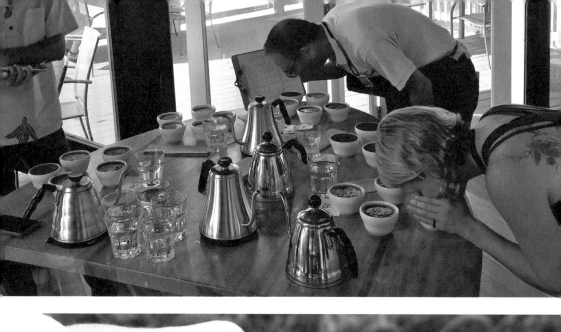

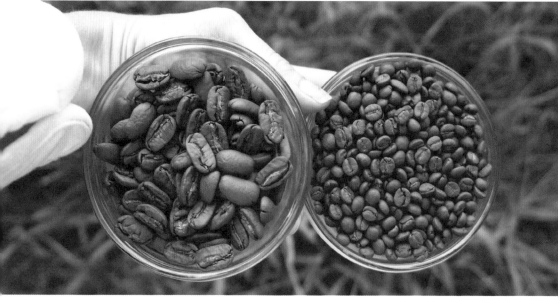

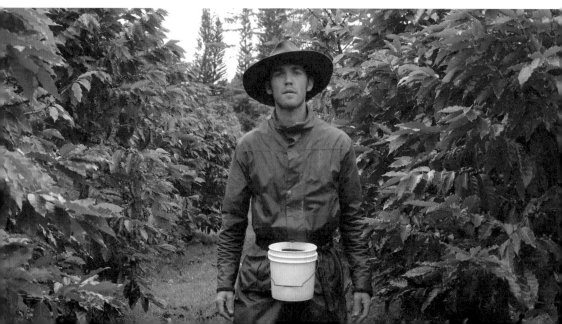

INNOVATION AND CHANGE

Embracing technology is part of the balance between innovation and tradition for us. Due to time restraints there are things that we have to cut corners on, but we do not want that to be the product. For example, we automate some of our emails and try to create better administration systems that require less thinking time. We can then use whatever 'random access memory' we have available to us to use for other things, such as strategy and problem-solving, to process and digest. We have become better at utilizing technology, using our time, and prioritizing, and we want to encourage others to do the same.

In food and coffee and farming we are in a situation where people earn very low wages and they can't make a sustainable living from it. Coffee is continuing to go through that crisis. We and everyone else have to think about how to make a living from it. For that reason, we very much feel like we are part of a larger group. When we first moved here and started doing what we do, the coffee scene was fairly dismal in Hawaii. Since then it has grown quite a bit. We have been a really active part of trying to grow speciality coffee here. We now have this base of people who are incredibly interested in how we are making coffee, and so it feels like even when there are a lot of hard days, and you want to just give it all up, there are people there that care. When the volcano erupted in 2018, people were texting us saying: 'Don't let the coffee go up in flames!' Even when situations seem desperate, you have other people rooting for you; it is like you are crowd-sourcing motivation.

MAINTAINING INTEGRITY

As producers, we do not want to have a big farm that mechanically harvests. We want to harvest by hand because you get more control over the quality of the fruit that you pick and that in turn gives you the foundation for the quality of the coffee. We don't want to compromise that process. That being said, lots of coffees are harvested mechanically and still taste good; it's just not something we have an interest in doing.

We are quite modern as coffee farmers go, especially in Hawaii. When people ask to buy a whole crop we say no because we have other customers and we don't want to sell out. If we increased supply it would feel less special and exclusive. There are some things that we want for our best customers – they are not necessarily the people who are willing to pay the most but they are often the people that have been with us the longest. If we mass-produce our products, they lose value in an emotional way. As the makers, we get to choose who gets our best products, and if that's the one thing we can control then we will. We don't always have time to be with our families and the people who have supported us but we can give the things that have taken our time. It is important to be true to yourself and your ethics.

FROM FARM TO CUP

01 Cultivation Like most orchard crops, coffee begins the cycle of fruit development shortly after the harvest is over. First, we prune the trees for desired stature, improved yield, and overall vigour. Then we feed throughout the season to produce healthy fruits. Quality begins here.

02 Harvest Coffee is a fruit, and we therefore treat it as such. Harvesting at peak ripeness ensures maximum sweetness, flavour, nuance, and balance is achieved. If poor fruits are selected, no amount or method of processing can improve the quality. Potential is determined by selective harvesting.

03 Processing Perhaps the most complicated step, 'processing' is a broad term describing the method used to prepare coffee for drying. A myriad of techniques range from drying the coffee fruit fully intact to implementing a fully washed process whereby the fruit and pulp are removed, leaving just the seeds to dry.

04 Drying Drying requires that coffee loses water at a particular rate. Too fast and the coffee loses sweetness, acidity, nuance, and shelf life; too slow and the coffee may taste mouldy, sour, or dirty. When properly executed, coffee tastes lovely for a long time.

05 'Resting'/Curing After most of the water leaves the coffee seed/bean, a period of 'rest' for sixty to ninety days is required to stabilize the water activity inside and allow for a consistent roasting process. During this time, the coffee cures in an environmentally controlled room.

06 Milling & grading Once cured, coffee must have one final layer of husk (known as 'parchment') removed before roasting. Then it is graded by size and density to remove physical defects and under-ripe seeds, resulting in a uniform size and appearance.

07 Roasting Arguably the most influential step in coffee's long journey, roasting brings the whole story to life for our senses. Art and science weave together to develop a wide range of experiences, from the comfort of familiarity to the excitement of exoticism.

08 Quality control: cupping Cupping is the process of formal evaluation where coffee is assessed for aroma, flavour, body, acidity, and aftertaste. Coffees are smelled and tasted side by side. Any problems or delightful surprises in the coffee will be found in this procedure.

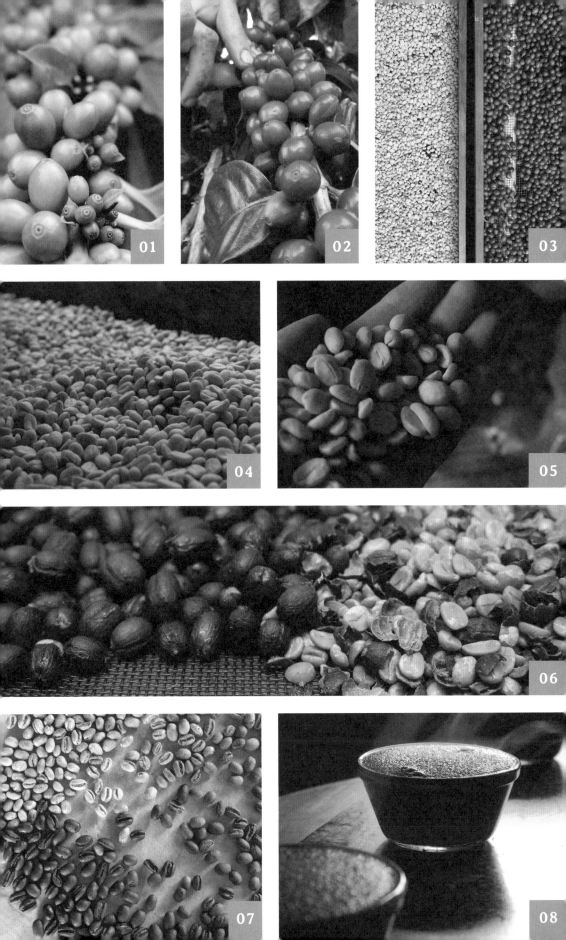

GROWING & FORAGING

Growing your own fruit and vegetables is something that a lot of people can try themselves – whether you have access to a garden, balcony with pots, allotment, or even a communal growing space. There is something wholesome about being able to nurture and pick the food that you put on the table. It offers a chance to reconnect with nature and an opportunity to be mindful. Much of it comes back to soil as a starting point, and the importance of looking after soil health. Hand-picking also offers a potentially more sustainable option than industrialized farming. In this section we meet proponents of no-dig gardening and heritage fruit alongside a botanicals forager, all of whom place great value on the beauty and self-sustaining attributes of nature. We also meet a slightly different type of forager based in Iceland who harnesses the minerals and energy around him to supply top chefs with high-quality sea salt.

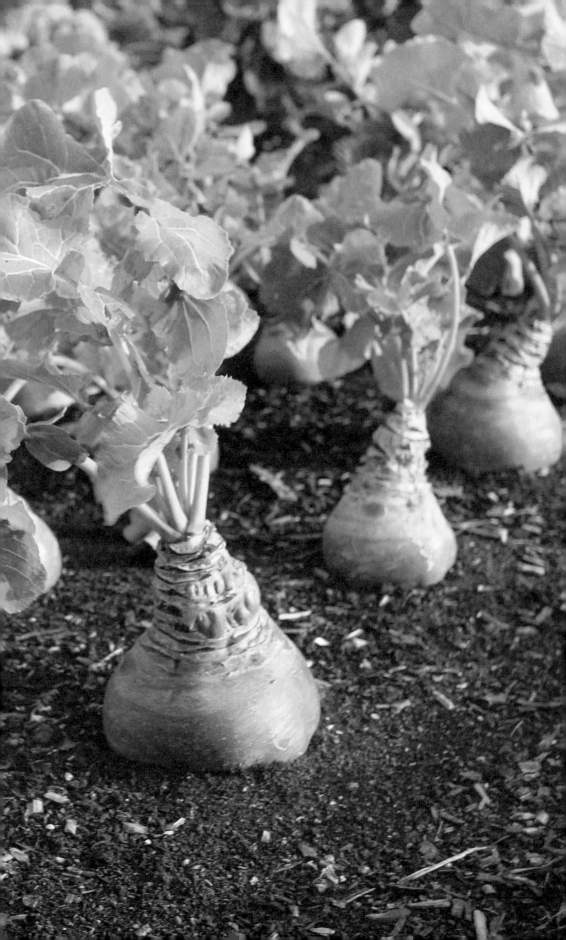

NO-DIG VEGETABLES

Vegetables come in all different shapes, sizes, colours, textures, and flavours. The option of buying 'wonky' vegetables in supermarkets is becoming a popular choice as opposed to only buying perfectly shaped carrots – after all, nature is not perfect and not all peppers and tomatoes need to be identical for us to enjoy their taste and nutrients. But what if you take it a step further and let nature really do its own thing by not interfering with the soil and not adding harmful pesticides and fertilizers to what we are consuming? No-dig follows these principles not only as a beautiful way of working with nature rather than trying to change it, but also as a mindful, time-saving, and potentially money-saving pastime in a fast-paced world.

"The beauty of compost-making is that
you are converting waste materials
into something really useful"

Charles Dowding

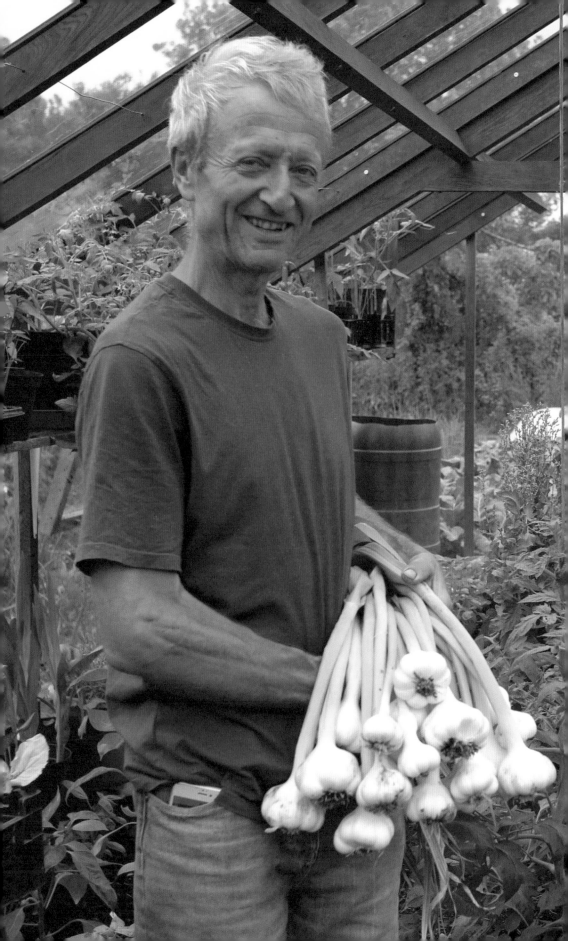

CHARLES DOWDING

MARKET GARDENER, AUTHOR & TEACHER

Somerset, UK | charlesdowding.co.uk

I grew up on a farm in the 1970s so I was quite intimately involved with farming at that time. I could see the use of fertilizers and synthetic chemical sprays for both dairy and cereals. Then at university I became interested in nutrition. That led me to wonder what was in food and what was on it in terms of chemical residues; I realized it maybe wasn't all as good as it seemed. I became interested in how soil works, what it consists of, and the living elements of soil – that was what really fascinated me more than anything. I came across the concept of 'no-dig' through a desire to only do what needs to be done and allow biological processes to occur as part of nature. I started off rotovating grass to kill the weeds in my garden and develop plant beds. Then I thought, 'I've got these lovely beds, why don't I just leave them?'

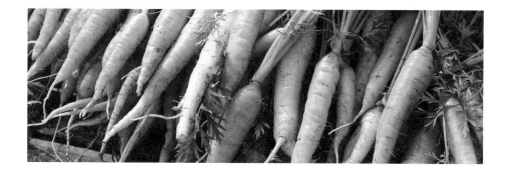

WHAT IS NO-DIG?

No-dig is a very simple method, but what you can learn from it is huge. It is actually just about encouraging nature and the natural processes to do their thing, by copying the environment and seeing how it works. With no-dig you are adding organic matter such as compost on top of the soil and leaving it, rather than turning the soil and adding the compost in. This encourages organisms such as worms to come up to the surface, eat it, and convert it; their excretions become food for other organisms and plant roots as well. There is then a whole series of other invisible natural processes occurring, such as the development of extensive networks of fungi.

"Everything links in and ties back to a simple starting point: don't disturb the soil, just feed it from the surface"

From my experience, including trials, I have found that any kind of disturbance of the soil that you find in other cultivation methods breaks up these networks, and plants end up not thriving quite so well. Fungi are really important in helping plant roots to access food and moisture. No-dig also allows soil to drain well, thanks to allowing a stable structure to develop. Everything links in and ties back to a simple starting point: don't disturb the soil, just feed it from the surface.

The detail occurs when you consider what kind of organic matter you are going to put on the surface to feed the soil life. There is nowhere in nature where goodness is dug or ploughed in. No-dig is very simple, but it is powered by an understanding of how soil and soil life work.

I ran a trial in two areas in my garden to compare growth using the same compost mulch in both. In one area I forked the soil to loosen it, with compost on the surface, and in the other area I added compost to the surface and left it 'no-dig'. In five years of cropping, we have recorded five per cent lower yields in the forked area. A by-product of not disturbing the soil is that carbon stays in the ground rather than being oxidized and converted to carbon dioxide. This reduces carbon dioxide in the air, improves drainage, and helps soil to hold more moisture and food.

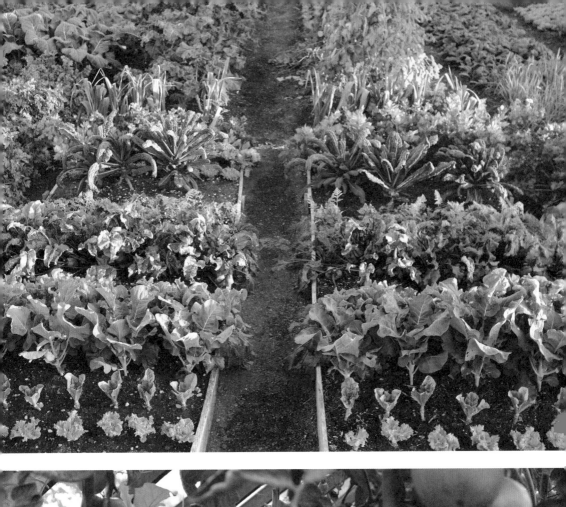

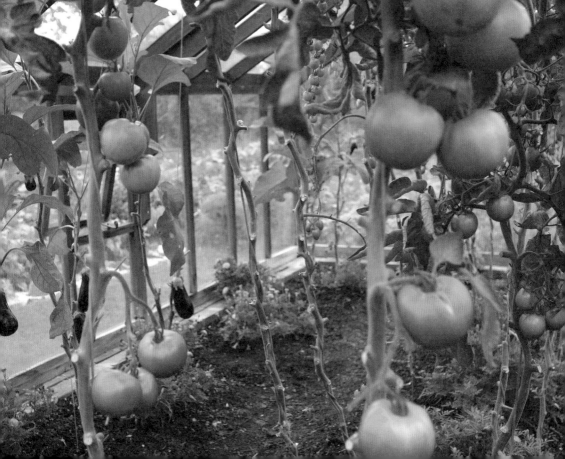

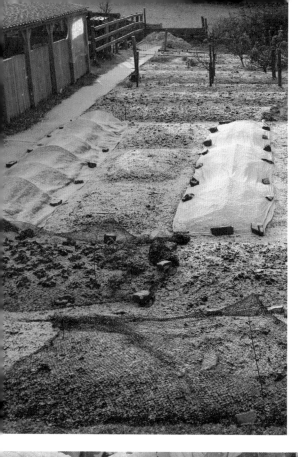

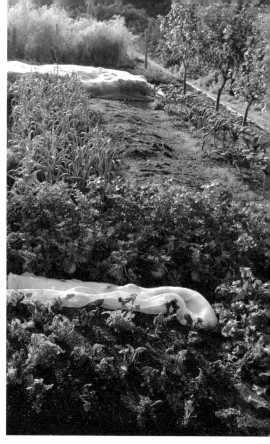

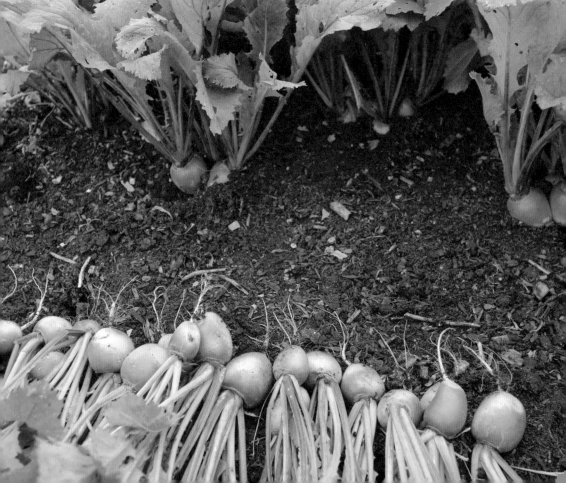

EXPLORING BENEATH THE SURFACE

For a long time, plant nutrition has been seen as being all about NPK (nitrogen, phosphorus, and potassium), nutrients, and fertilizers, where you have what are called 'heavy-feeding plants' and 'light-feeding plants'. The implicit assumption is that plants' roots are like mouths waiting to gulp down the nutrients you give them in whatever form. It turns out that this is not actually the case. I think throughout farming there has been a misunderstanding of how plants actually grow and the importance of fungal interactions. The fungi attach their network to plant roots and help them find nutrients and moisture. They are very small and can creep into minuscule crevices in the soil to extract food and water that plant roots can't access. This is where no-dig and no-till really win; they are not disturbing the fungal networks, which means plants are well fed without the gardener needing to worry about giving food to plants because the fungi are organized to find it. In return, plant roots feed the fungi with carbon energy powered by photosynthesis. These bits of knowledge give you a sense of the importance of doing less and leaving soil alone; it is just working out *how* you do that.

> "I think throughout farming there has been misunderstanding of how plants actually grow and the importance of fungal interactions"

Another reason that no-dig works is that if you are not rotovating, digging, or disturbing the soil, you are not exposing it to air, which means that moisture is conserved. Also, when it rains on preserved, undamaged soil structure, the rain soaks in better and doesn't wash off so easily. You therefore get more value from summer storms and less flooding.

I have tested this principle using two beds side-by-side – one dig and one no-dig. When demonstrating this experiment to people, I grow the same vegetables and use the same amount of compost in each one, yet the visual contrasts between the two is always so interesting. In the trial, we took photographs while pouring twenty-five litres of water on each bed. On the no-dig bed with a compost mulch, you see how the water just disappears downwards; whereas on the dig bed where you have soil on top, the water just puddles because the fine particles of dug soil stick together. Very quickly these particles form a surface layer of dense, impenetrable material, a sort of clay, and the rest of the water drains away from the plant rather than into the soil. If you consider the implications of that for fields that are ploughed and then subjected to heavy thunderstorms and flooding, the ramifications are huge. It is incredible that just with this simple piece of knowledge, this simple trial, you can witness and understand what is happening.

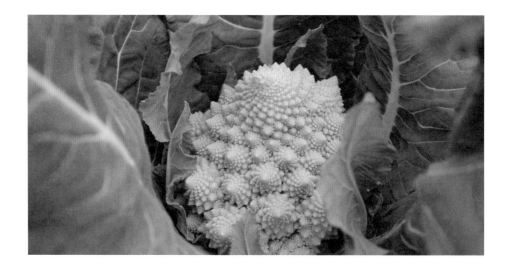

NUTRITION

I became interested in the health benefits of no-dig vegetables when I joined the Soil Association in 1981. They look at links between the health of soil, the health of plants, the health of animals, and the health of people. This also relates to the knowledge that is emerging now about nutrition and soil quality. Suddenly people are realizing how important the gut is and that the gut needs microbes to function properly. And guess what? They are the same microbes you have in healthy soil. It is difficult to find such a resource if you live in the middle of a city, although you could find an allotment and build up the soil life there. That is where no-dig is really powerful. You are creating healthy soil full of these great microbes – a wonderful health resource right in your own garden.

"We are now starting to see more of an encouragement of proactive health and well-being"

This concept of nutrition having a relationship with soil organisms is something I really want to promote. Even growers and farmers using organic principles sometimes lost sight of the fragility of living soil. For example, until recently for many people the term 'organic' had become about avoiding synthetic chemicals, and there wasn't emphasis on the positive side, which is soil health and vitality. This links to a whole different way of looking at health and disease, which is that health is a positive state, not just an absence of disease. I think we are now starting to see more of an encouragement of proactive health and well-being, which is a positive step.

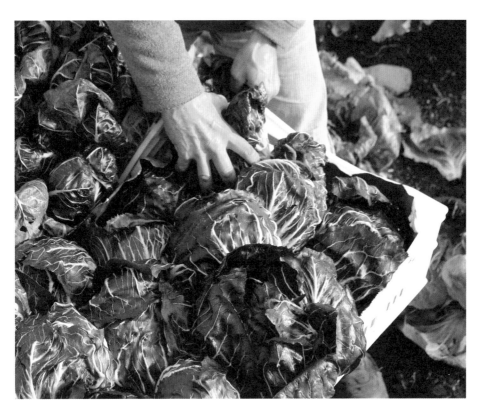

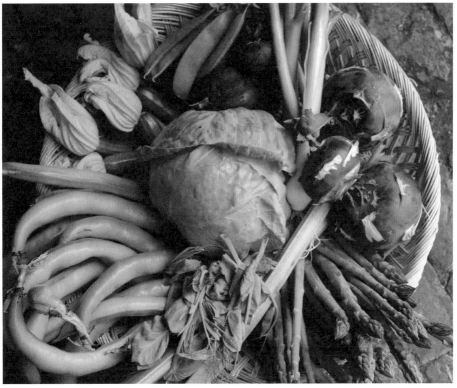

NO-DIG: TIPS & BASIC PRINCIPLES

Small is plenty

Even one bed measuring 1.2 × 2.4 m can grow a lot of food. Cropping a small area and keeping it full is more productive and fun than having weeds and empty spaces in a larger area.

Start as you mean to go on

There is no need to dig first, or fork, because plants root better in dense, firm soil than when the structure is loose and offers less support. No-dig works well on clay soil when you maintain a surface mulch of organic matter. You can plant or sow immediately into a mulch of compost.

Dealing with weeds

How you kill weeds when starting no-dig depends on which weeds you have, how many there are, and how much organic matter you can source. If you have small weeds, a mulch (surface application) of 5 cm of compost can clear them by light deprivation; the compost mulch also feeds soil organisms.

You may have weeds or plants that need digging out initially. Docks and woody plants such as brambles are best removed with a sharp spade before mulching, otherwise they push mulches up

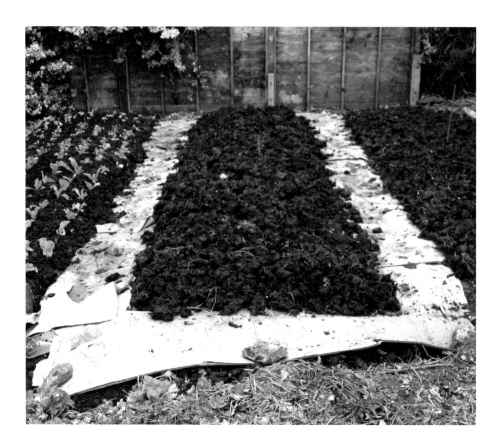

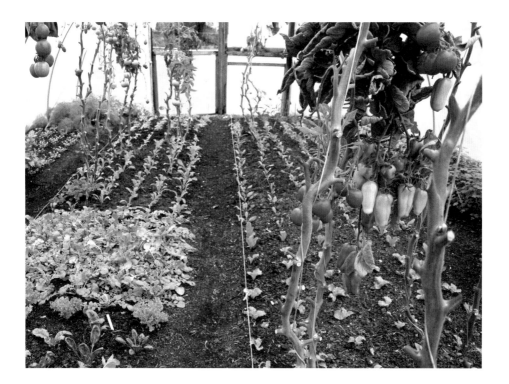

and reach light before they die. Use a sharp spade to cut around bramble clumps, removing the main crown but leaving small roots in the soil so that they feed microbes when decomposing, and also to reduce soil disturbance.

Aim for weed-free paths. Thick cardboard is effective, perhaps held down with just a thin covering of woody mulch. If weeds grow through, lay more cardboard on top. Repeat this process two months later if weeds still grow. You can even simply plant on top of cardboard-covered beds by adding 15 cm of compost on top of the cardboard.

Wooden sides
It is often assumed that growing in beds means you need permanent sides, but this is untrue, though they are sometimes useful the first few months to keep compost-filled beds in shape.

Tip for slugs
Gardens are difficult for vegetables if there are many hiding places for slugs – shady areas, bits of long grass, or shrubs and bushes drooping onto the ground. These provide the moist, dark habitat that is basically a slug's home. If possible, grow your vegetables as far away as possible from those kinds of places. Also, keep your garden as tidy as possible. In some ways this contradicts the idea of giving nature a free hand – but the ordered way in which we tend to grow vegetables is not natural. As you wander through a forest you won't see a bed of lettuce or a row of carrots; however, you can maintain your growth in a natural way and avoid using pesticides.

SOURCING COMPOST

Compost is anything decomposed, including animal manures, leaf mould, and woody wastes. People ask how they can afford enough compost. My reply to that is that no-dig doesn't need more compost than if you were digging or cultivating. It is simply that it is using it more efficiently and more obviously on the surface. Also I encourage people to crop a smaller area and do it more intensively, which means in the end you don't require so much compost.

Organic matter for growing can be so many different things and varies geographically. In very dry climates, for example, the organic matter most appropriate is often dry grass and straw, which can just sit on top of the surface. If you do that in the UK, however, you attract slugs, because here our climate is much damper, so undecomposed organic matter on the surface serves as a habitat for creatures you don't want. In the UK, the organic matter I use is anything decomposed. It needs to be reasonably well decomposed but it doesn't have to be perfect – a few slightly woody components are fine. I aim to cover my beds with compost by year-end, so that it protects soil over winter and is a food source for soil organisms, which slowly take it into the soil. You end up with a soft, dark surface that is simple to sow into.

The beauty of compost-making is that you are converting waste materials into something really useful, so it is a question of whatever you can get hold of. You can start with your own waste: any organic matter from your household, vegetable peelings, even a bit of wood ash from a fire, whatever you might have – even scrunched-up newspaper is great. It is all good. The key thing is to achieve proportions of roughly half green and fresh, and half older and brown. There is a bit more to it than that but this works as a broad outline.

"People love it in terms of feeling a deeper connection with natural processes and seeing those living transformations at work"

Another benefit of making your own compost is that you can convert other people's waste too, so you can do a service to your community. For example, there is a lot of coffee waste, and that can be really valuable for the compost heap. It is quite rich and raw, so it is better to put it in the compost heap than on your soil, but it helps everything else to break down, and you end up with more compost. I am really working to get the information out there about making your own compost. Not only is it a practical, useful thing, it is actually quite a spiritual thing to do. I have noticed people love it in terms of feeling a deeper connection with natural processes and seeing those living transformations at work.

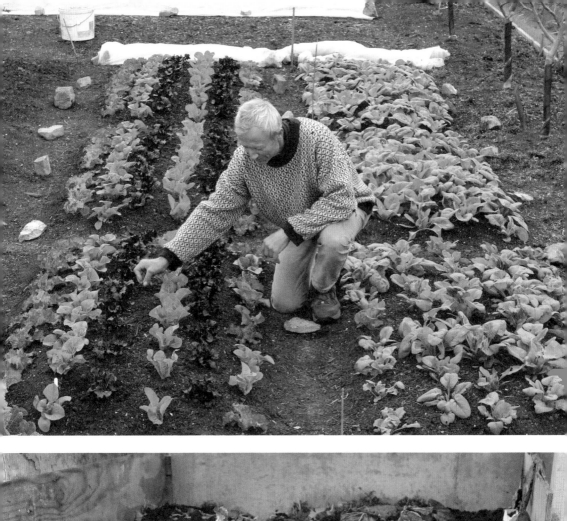

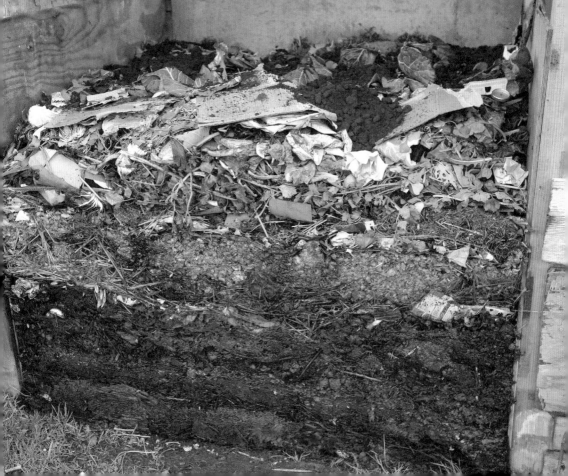

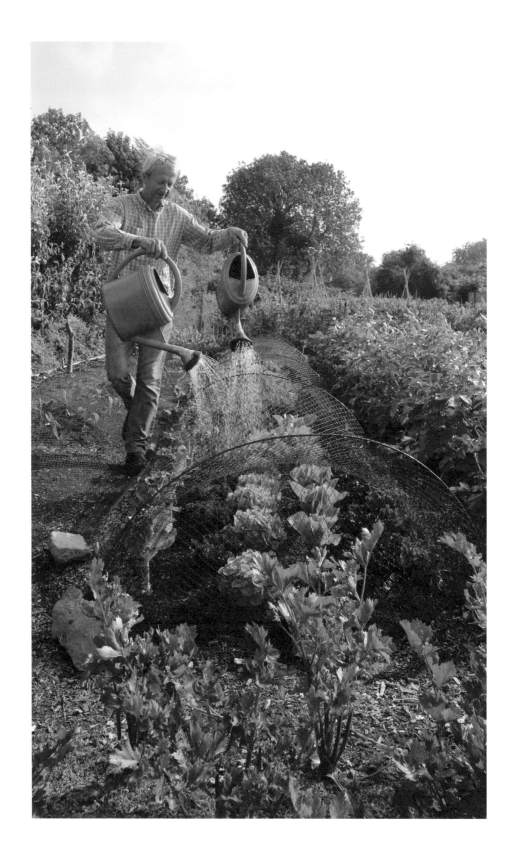

CULTIVATING A CAREER

If you are thinking about developing a career in something like gardening, you have to build up your experience. In my case I have been fortunate, but it's not easy to make a living from simple gardening. For a beginner, particularly if you are selling vegetables through market-gardening, you need supplementary income or a day job.

I have a market garden from which I sell over £20,000 of vegetables a year. My garden work is about thirty-five hours a week in the summer, and I employ people doing about the same amount to achieve that revenue. We have been selling bags of salad leaves because they are effectively the highest-value product. We couldn't make a living selling bunches of carrots or beetroots, but with salad leaves it is possible.

I don't sell at actual markets now at all because they take too much time, especially in the UK where there isn't that market culture where people rely on them. Instead, I sell pre-ordered vegetables to local outlets such as restaurants, pubs, and shops. They send me an order twice a week and I fulfil it. This way I know roughly what they are going to request so there is less waste and very little time lost; it also means you develop a strong relationship with them. Professionalism and remaining reliable with the growing side of things are important. Customers know my produce is going be there when they need it.

The margins are very tight to make a profit at this however, which means you have a very small amount of profit to pay a wage. You have therefore got to be very efficient, which is where no-dig really works. Fewer weeds means you are not wasting time weeding, and you can get on with the more important things that produce revenue. I think we are seeing a bit of a revolution in growing and gardening as more people realize this.

It is the courses I run that are the pinnacle in terms of earning possibility. Writing is somewhere in the middle in terms of income. I also earn some money from videos online if people click on the third-party advertisements.

The interesting thing is that I have almost never advertised. It all happens through word of mouth and my website, so the reputation just develops. That said, I think the two things that have probably made the biggest difference to me in terms of getting my name out there are national television and writing a book. Again, I was fortunate; I was just gardening in my seven-acre garden (in those days it was quite large) and someone hopped over the fence from the road. It turned out that he was the producer of the BBC's *Gardener's World* programme. This was the late 1980s and he asked how I would feel if they came and did some filming. I said yes and it just went from there.

PRIORITIZING EDUCATION

My work with media of all types has propelled my reputation and helped me to reach a wider audience. Through my courses, books, and online resources I can inform people and give them an understanding that empowers them. It is good for people to question things and understand the science behind them. They can then build on that comprehension and apply it to their own situations. I don't look to give people a formula – how to do this and how to do that in every situation – but a grounding so that they can choose and use slightly different methods; the beauty of gardening is that every garden is different.

I ensure my website is packed with information about things I have learned. I am very happy if people then book my courses as a result, but I don't want to keep information hidden from people as a marketing tool. One of the lovely things about gardening and growing is that there is actually no end to what you can learn, so there is always more to find out. I love sharing what I have learned because I really want people to succeed. I think growing your own food and experiencing the pleasure of both growing it, and eating something you have grown, is a very worthwhile aim for people.

I also find that YouTube is a really powerful tool for reaching out to people all over the world. Once you reach a certain number of subscribers, some social media channels will promote you further, which then means you can reach an even larger audience. In 2018, I won the Garden Media Guild Social Media Influencer of the Year award, which was fantastic. I really like the fact that people enjoy watching gardening videos.

NATURE'S TRADITION AS REVOLUTIONARY

Simple as it may be, no-dig is actually revolutionary. It contradicts most traditional teaching. But you can't just expect someone to buy into it straightaway. I have been called things like 'lazy' because I wasn't doing a proper job and 'wasn't exerting myself'. Now, I am starting to hear that a lot less. No-dig has crossed the threshold of social acceptance.

While some of the crafts in this book reinforce tradition, because traditional methods often have a lot to offer in terms of sustainability, no-dig bucks that trend. Oddly enough, I would say the tradition of digging and quite a few traditions in gardening need to be reconsidered. Examples include crop rotation, hardening off, and watering in sunlight. The commonly prescribed methods tend to waste people's time. Traditions should not become crystallized and immovable. They can inform and be a good starting point, but then we need to learn how to improve on that with modern materials or technology, and new understandings. There needs to be a readiness to review what a tradition is based on and to examine it in the current context – as many of the innovators in this book do.

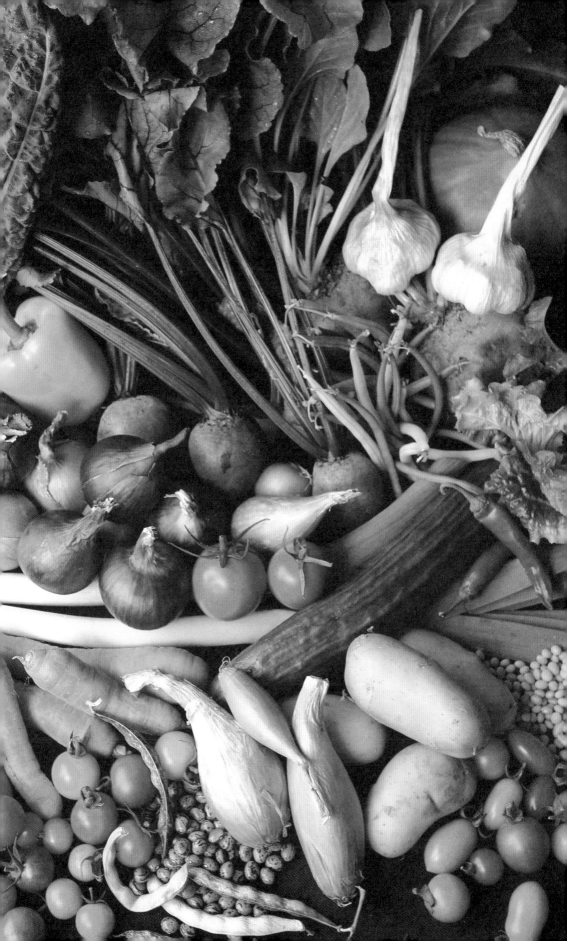

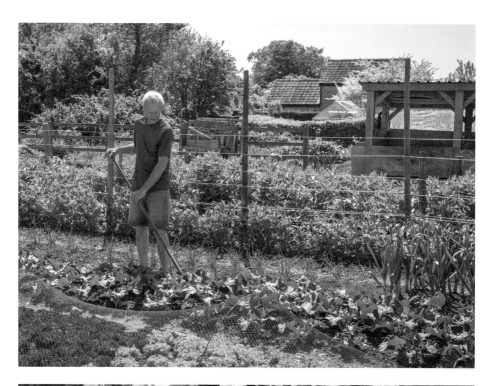

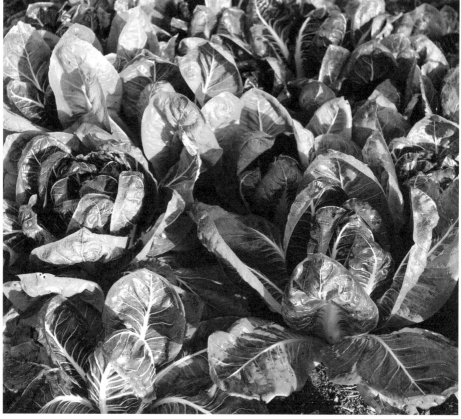

GROWING YOUR OWN – AND BEYOND

Most of the market gardeners I know who use organic methods only compare notes with other market gardeners who use organic methods; they are not really talking to recreational gardeners, and vice versa. However, these two areas of cultivation overlap, and the no-dig methods I use are equally applicable whether you are a home gardener or a market gardener. Spanning the two puts me in a strong position to share information more widely. I seek to bridge the gap, and it is empowering for people because it takes away that notion that food has to be produced by professionals.

There are many people who are in an in-between place with professional market gardening and recreational gardening – they are selling some produce but they also have other sources of income. I give a lot of advice to people who are doing small-scale selling just to their local community. They earn some pocket money at least, and the local people get lovely fresh food. This whole middle ground is growing, and that is exciting because it ticks so many sustainability boxes: freshness of produce, bringing people together, and reducing transport costs and unnecessary packaging. I think growing your own is a really important option that could be utilized more. Home producers can actually produce a lot of food.

"It is empowering for people because it takes away that notion that food has to be produced by professionals"

THE BEAUTY OF EFFICIENCY

One of the things I enjoy the most about no-dig is the efficiency. No-dig results in much fewer weeds and that offers an idea of how healthy the soil is. In my experience, weeds grow where soil is disturbed. They are part of a recovery mechanism, so when you don't see weeds it is a really good sign that you know that things are okay. The thing that I love about the no-dig method, therefore, is how it frees you up. I have time to be creative and plant and harvest and make the garden attractive, while appreciating the sheer beauty of vegetables and allowing nature to express itself, as far as is possible in vegetable growing. When you understand and embrace the potential of soil and how plants grow, vegetables can be dazzling. This is important because it draws the gardener in more to experience the beauty, and then also to harvest it.

I feel extremely fortunate because I can combine the physical activity of gardening with other administration and media activities, which are equally important in my work. I encourage everybody who has a bit of ground nearby to take it on and get involved, and also not to withdraw too much in the winter. It is good to be outside in these months to absorb more light, and obviously it gets you moving, plus your garden will benefit. Gardening is rewarding and health-giving.

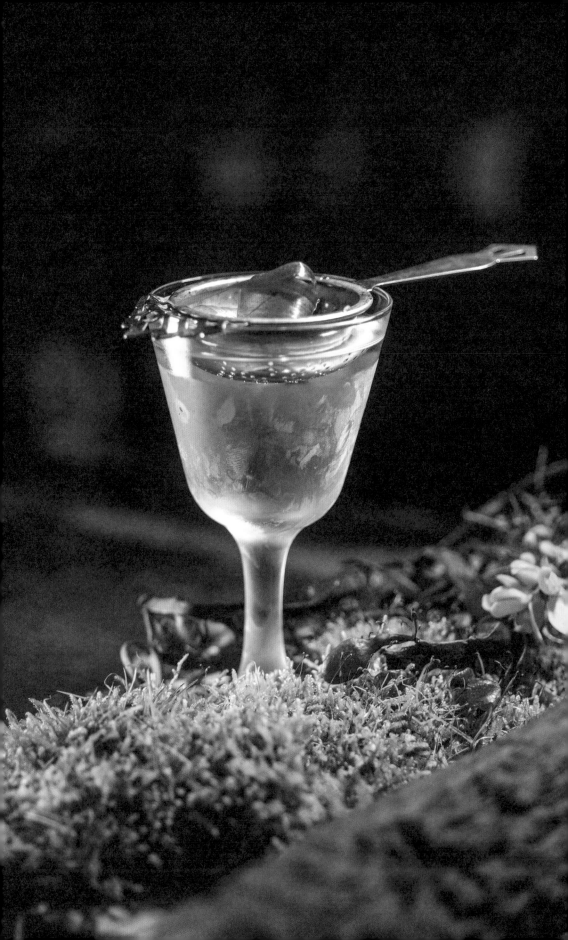

GIN

With its juniper berry base and astonishingly wide range of natural aromatic botanicals, gin is one of the most diversely blended alcoholic spirits, and is a key ingredient of many classic cocktails. Traditionally served over ice with (increasingly sophisticated) variations of tonic water, gin makes a refreshing highball cocktail – especially popular in the summer months.

A quintessentially English drink, gin has notable fans, including Noël Coward, Charles Dickens, Jay Gatsby, and Dorothy Parker. Its popularity has soared in recent years, as makers have experimented with flavoured variations, and mass-market producers and small craft businesses have been competing for a share of the expanding market.

"The taste is rich and mellow, cool on entry then warming across the palate, stimulating the taste buds with a round mouthfeel and citrus freshness"

Adam Hannett, Head Distiller, Bruichladdich Distillery

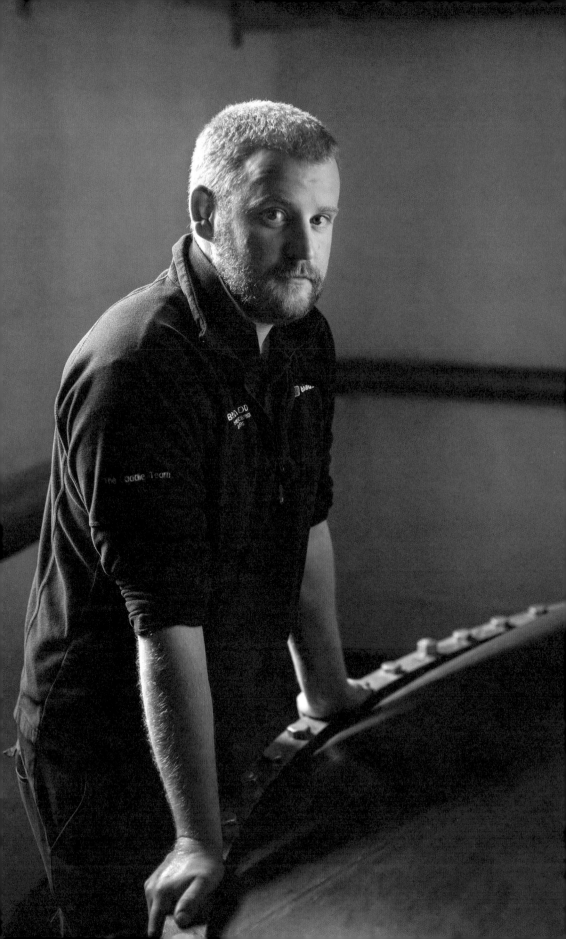

BRUICHLADDICH DISTILLERY

Islay, Scotland | bruichladdich.com

While Bruichladdich is traditionally a whisky distillery, this chapter will focus on its mould-breaking gin, The Botanist. The Botanist came to life in 2010 after a meeting of minds and serendipitous circumstances on the Isle of Islay in the Southern Hebrides in Scotland.

Through boom and bust times, Bruichladdich Distillery has changed through many hands in the industry. In 1994 it was forced to close its doors due to industry pressures; many thought for good. It was rescued in 2004 by Mark Reynier and Simon Coughlin, fine-wine merchants from London. Fascinated by the concept of terroir, they wanted to create spirits which spoke of the land they were from. Alongside the surviving Victorian equipment and traditional methods, they implemented a progressive, convention-challenging attitude; these visionaries wanted to make whisky in the traditional way, employing real people with long-held skills.

Time moved on and the distillery became a greater and greater success, with more stale industry boundaries being challenged. As an example, many whiskies claim to be 'Islay whisky' but in reality they are distilled here from ingredients that don't come from the island. They are then shipped off the island to be matured in casks on the mainland, spending the absolute minimum amount of time on Islay. We aim to be a true island business as much as possible.

Never shy of a new venture – and partial to a gin and tonic – Mark and Simon, alongside Bruichladdich's Master Distiller Jim McEwan and Distillery Manager Duncan McGillivray, conceived a gin inspired by, and created with, botanicals from Islay.

Jim sought advice from two professional botanists, Dr Richard Gulliver and Mrs Mavis Gulliver, who at the time lived in Port Ellen on Islay. Richard and Mavis introduced Jim to around thirty-three herbs, leaves, and flowers that could be foraged sustainably on the island and provided a wide range of scents and flavours. Through a process of olfactory experimentation and elimination, Jim proposed a balanced recipe of twenty-two Islay botanicals. This is the same recipe used today, testament to the skills and dedication of the original team.

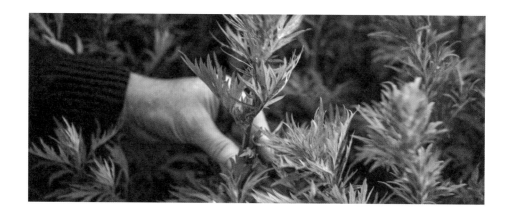

WILD

'Wild, foraged, distilled' is how we describe The Botanist, a gin born of its island home, Islay, a small Hebridean island on the far west of Scotland. It is a cliché perhaps of windswept shores and heather moors, but life here doesn't allow all the comforts and ease of the mainland living. 'Wild' nods to the nature of Bruichladdich and the people who make this spirit. It is a fiercely independent distillery and when the gin was conceived, it broke the mould at the time. The 'gin boom' was yet to happen. A whisky distillery with already matured stock making a gin? Why? Because we could. It was part of our evolution as distillers, and it is in our DNA to try new things and push industry boundaries.

THE IMPORTANCE OF TERROIR

The Botanist gin is a story of place, a rare expression of the heart and soul of Islay. We think locality and terroir matters. In the world of fine wine, terroir is a concept that reflects the inter-action of soil, subsoil, exposure, orientation, climate, and microclimate on the growth of the vine and the harvest of the grape. At Bruichladdich, we believe terroir is vital. We believe it imparts subtle nuance and variety to sensory experience. It will have an effect on any food or drink. The more complex the flavours inherent in that food or drink, the more profound the effect.

When distilling The Botanist, we are creating something more than a drink. The Botanist is a representation of the place we are from. It is a way of communicating our place in the world and our love for it. We use the art of distillation and a connection to the land, our home, to create a wonderful spirit that speaks of the place it is from. The taste is rich and mellow, cool on entry then warming across the palate, stimulating the taste buds with a round mouthfeel and citrus freshness. This is a bewitching, delectable, and luxurious gin: its citrus freshness excites and stimulates the taste buds, allowing you to experience a starburst of flavours as they explode across the palate.

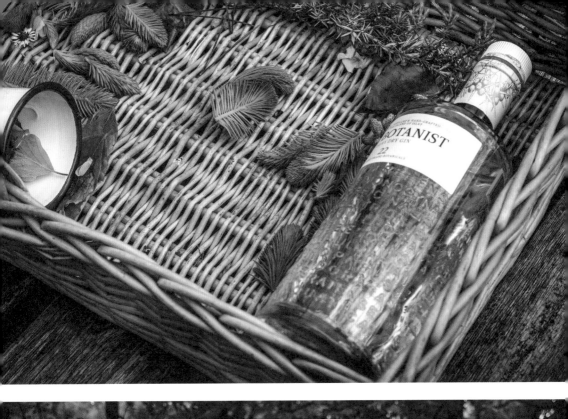

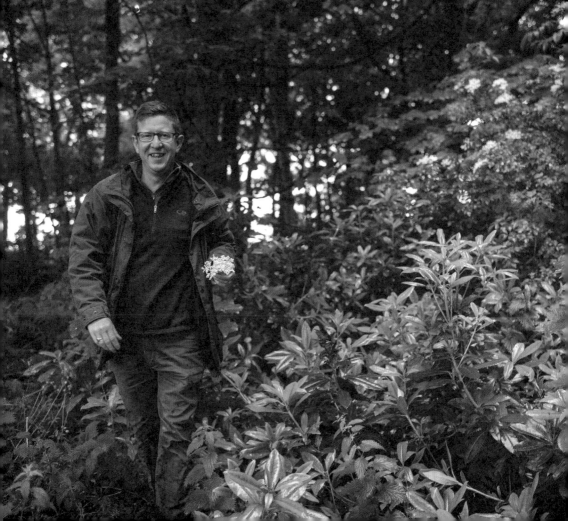

FORAGED

The Botanist's twenty-two Islay botanicals are sustainably hand-picked on the island by our own dedicated full-time forager, James Donaldson. Islay was always to be at the heart of the creation of The Botanist – its flavour, its people, and its sustainability.

James is our first full-time forager, and lives on Islay. He developed his love of the outdoors at a young age while exploring the parks and hedgerows of his home in Angus. He says it was then that he discovered his 'natural talent for falling in burns (bodies of water such as streams) and getting covered in mud.' After studying Botany at Edinburgh University, James spent time travelling but eventually returned to Scotland to take up a job as a tour guide. It was fate when the job as a Professional Forager was advertised at Bruichladdich, and James now says he is 'living the dream' in his role.

"We never take more than we need by carefully managing the amount of botanicals we pick to correspond with the amount of gin we produce"

When James joined The Botanist team in 2017, he spent the first six months of his time with our original botanists, Richard and Mavis. They passed on their knowledge of their previous methods of collection, preservation, and preparation of 'the twenty-two' to James. Richard and Mavis were retiring after spending ten years on the project, initially on the development of The Botanist, and then latterly foraging for distillations. Without this essential skill-sharing, we could not have continued to make our gin to the same standard.

Picking season begins in March when the gorse is in full bloom. Between March and September, processions of plants make their appearance on various parts of the island. Some grow for the entirety of this period; others, like hawthorn, make a very short appearance and have to be collected quickly over the course of one week. The botanicals are picked sustainably – we never take more than we need by carefully managing the amount of botanicals we pick to correspond with the amount of gin we produce. In addition to sustainable picking, we deliberately have not chosen any plants that are rare or threatened to make up our twenty-two botanicals.

In each distillation of The Botanist, a nominal amount of Islay juniper is added. Local juniper has all but been wiped out on the island, but we have embarked on a project to plant it back in. It is a favourite of the many sheep and wild goats that live on Islay, and was also used historically to fire illicit stills. We add a symbolic amount to our distillation to celebrate its heritage. In winter, James takes cuttings of the few remaining established plants, tends them for two to three years, and then replants them with the aim of establishing colonies. Last year he planted forty-eight young juniper plants.

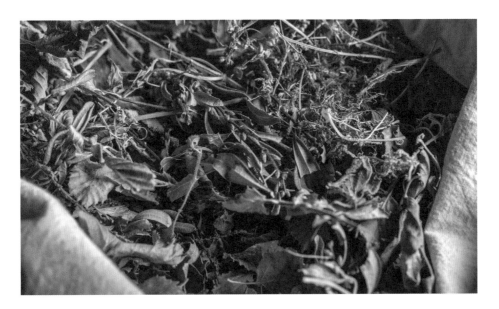

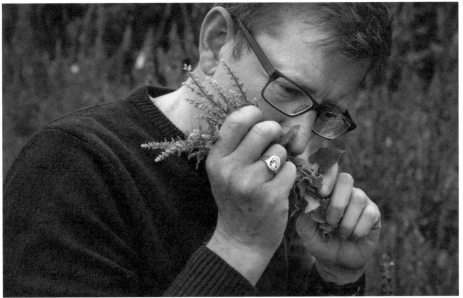

THE BOTANIST FOUNDATION

Bruichladdich Distillery runs The Botanist Foundation, which contributes to helping biodiversity and social causes. Over the last few years, we have been involved in a host of projects, including conservation, sustainability, pollination, local wildlife support, and environmental initiatives. For example, we work to improve the biodiversity on the distillery sites on Islay, have supported the Islay Natural History Trust with its compilation of a biological records database, and sponsor local pollinator projects.

DISTILLED

The Botanist comes from a home that had been distilling whisky for over 120 years before this new inception. The historic knowledge of distillation methods, including slow-trickle distillation to maintain oils and flavour in the spirit, alongside innovation by using multiple infusion methods upon the botanicals, was integral to the development of the gin process and meant that The Botanist was a truly unique creation.

When we created the initial concept of The Botanist we had no idea that it would become as popular as it has. As demand has grown, we have increased the number of distillations we do every year. But we in no way compromise on the recipe or production methods. Yes, we need to pick more island botanicals as a result, but we ensure that this is always done within the limits of it remaining sustainable. The process is still all carried out by hand using traditional methods – we just do more than we used to. Over the years the bottling hall at the distillery has grown from a four-bottle hand filler to full production lines accommodating both the whisky and the gin. The Botanist now has its own dedicated bottling line and this means more locals are employed here.

It is important to strike a balance between innovation and modernization and using small-scale traditional techniques. We distil our gin in an old Lomond still that has been radically modified to suit. The idea was to steep the bulk of the botanicals in the body of the still and then conduct a distillation at very low pressure, subjecting the vapours to maximum cleansing through contact with the copper. This ensures that only the lightest, purest vapours ever reach the island botanicals, held in a newly added bespoke casket in the lyne arm, prior to their reaching the condenser (the lyne arm links the head of the still to the condensing system – see p. 207). This is why our gin takes seventeen hours to distil – considerably longer than the average of six hours.

UGLY BETTY

Before The Botanist was developed, the distillery had acquired an old, rare Lomond still (a key piece of distillation apparatus) from a Dumbarton distillery about to be demolished. What was bought as spares to fix an ageing Victorian distillery contained a diamond in the rough – our gin still 'Ugly Betty', which you can see in the photographs at the top of the opposite page. Manager Duncan saw that what was one man's scrap was another's gold. After some heavy-duty modifications by Duncan and his team, she was ready to distil.

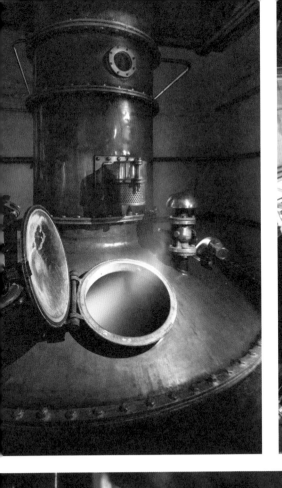
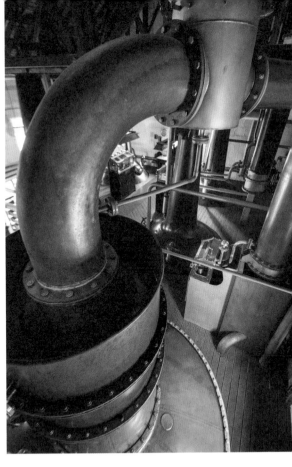
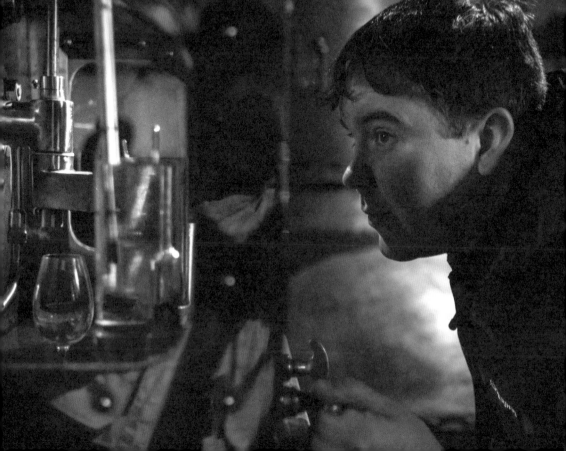

THE GIN-MAKING PROCESS

After foraging, James carefully lays out the botanicals in a special room to dry them. This preserves their flavour and aroma. Once they are dried, the botanicals are measured out in weight and the correct balance is added to unbleached calico bags.

01 MACERATION

Our gin is distilled in autumn and winter. One hundred per cent wheat grain spirit at ninety-six per cent diluted to fifty-seven percent using Islay spring water is added into the **base**. The core botanicals (roots, barks, peels, berries, and seed categories) are then manually loaded into the pot of the still in a particular order, and spread using rakes to form a sort of mat that sits on the surface of the liquid. They are then steeped for twelve hours.

02 DISTILLATION

The steam pressure is increased to simmering point for ten hours and the vapours start to rise up the **neck** of the heavily modified vessel. The rising vapours first hit a cluster of seventy-five small bore copper pipes in the neck that provide a massively increased surface area of copper, a powerful cleansing agent. They then hit a water box at the head of the still that cools the vapours and causes a reflux of any heavy oils that have escaped the copper.

Only the purest and lightest vapours turn through ninety degrees and enter the **lyne arm**, into which the casket containing the Islay botanicals is built. The island botanicals are held in the unbleached calico bags through which the vapour can easily pass, but even at this stage there is a reflux pipe that returns any heavier condensed spirit to the neck of the still where it can be redistilled.

The final stage of the journey is down the long shell tube condenser and into The Botanist's own unique **spirit safe**, from which the stillman takes samples to determine the precious middle cut.[14] The process takes seventeen hours, which is achingly slow for gin.

03 BOTTLING

The middle cut is then mixed with the purest Islay spring water from Octomore Farm down to forty-six per cent, before being bottled on site in our bottling hall.

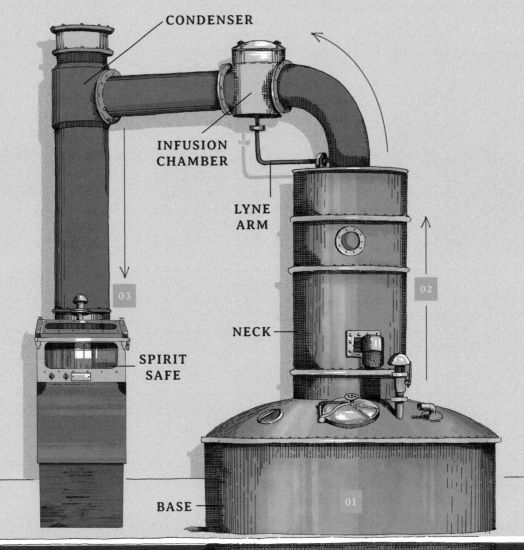

CONDENSER

INFUSION
CHAMBER

LYNE
ARM

03

SPIRIT
SAFE

NECK

02

BASE

01

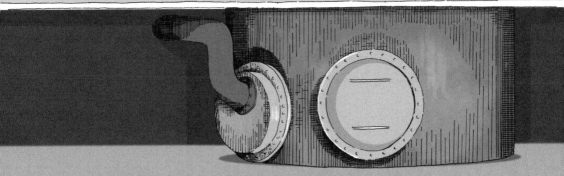

A HERITAGE MAINTAINED

Our Head Distiller, Adam Hannett, is now ultimately responsible for the quality of spirits at Bruichladdich, including The Botanist. However, twelve years ago when he was starting out, Adam was part of the tour guide team welcoming visitors to the old Victorian distillery. He enjoyed sharing the knowledge gained from the craftsmen he was working with and soon became fascinated with how they create and control the finest flavours in their spirits.

Adam's infectious enthusiasm and hard-working ethos was encouraged by the then Master Distiller, Jim McEwan. Recognizing Adam's remarkable nose and palate, Jim quickly invited Adam to work alongside him. Jim has now retired and Adam has seamlessly assumed the role his mentor prepared him for. Both Adam and James are forging their own way in the story of The Botanist, and they too will pass their skills on to the next generation of foragers and distillers.

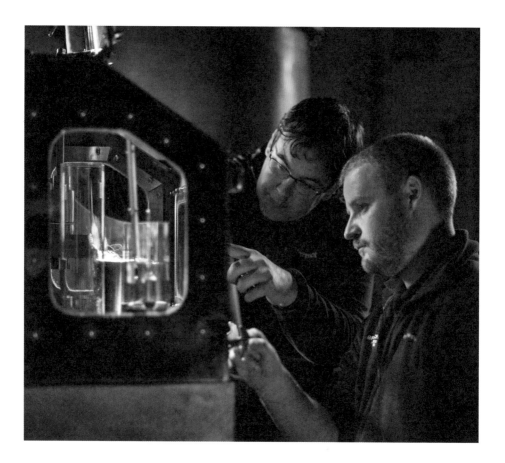

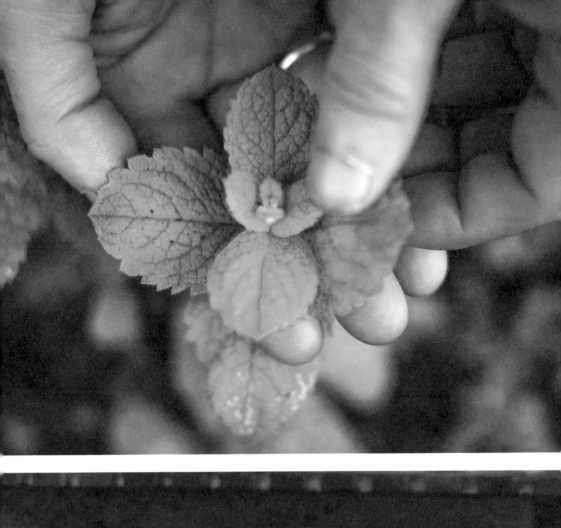
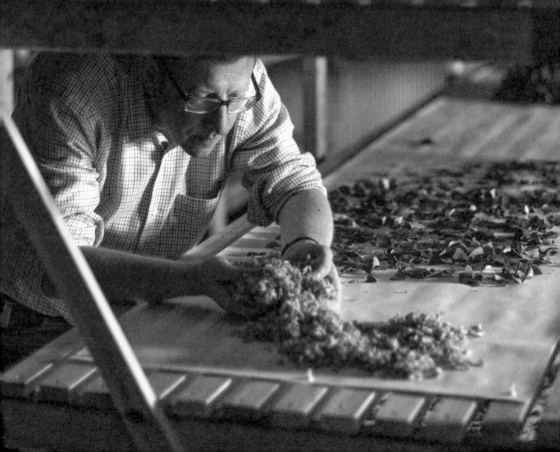

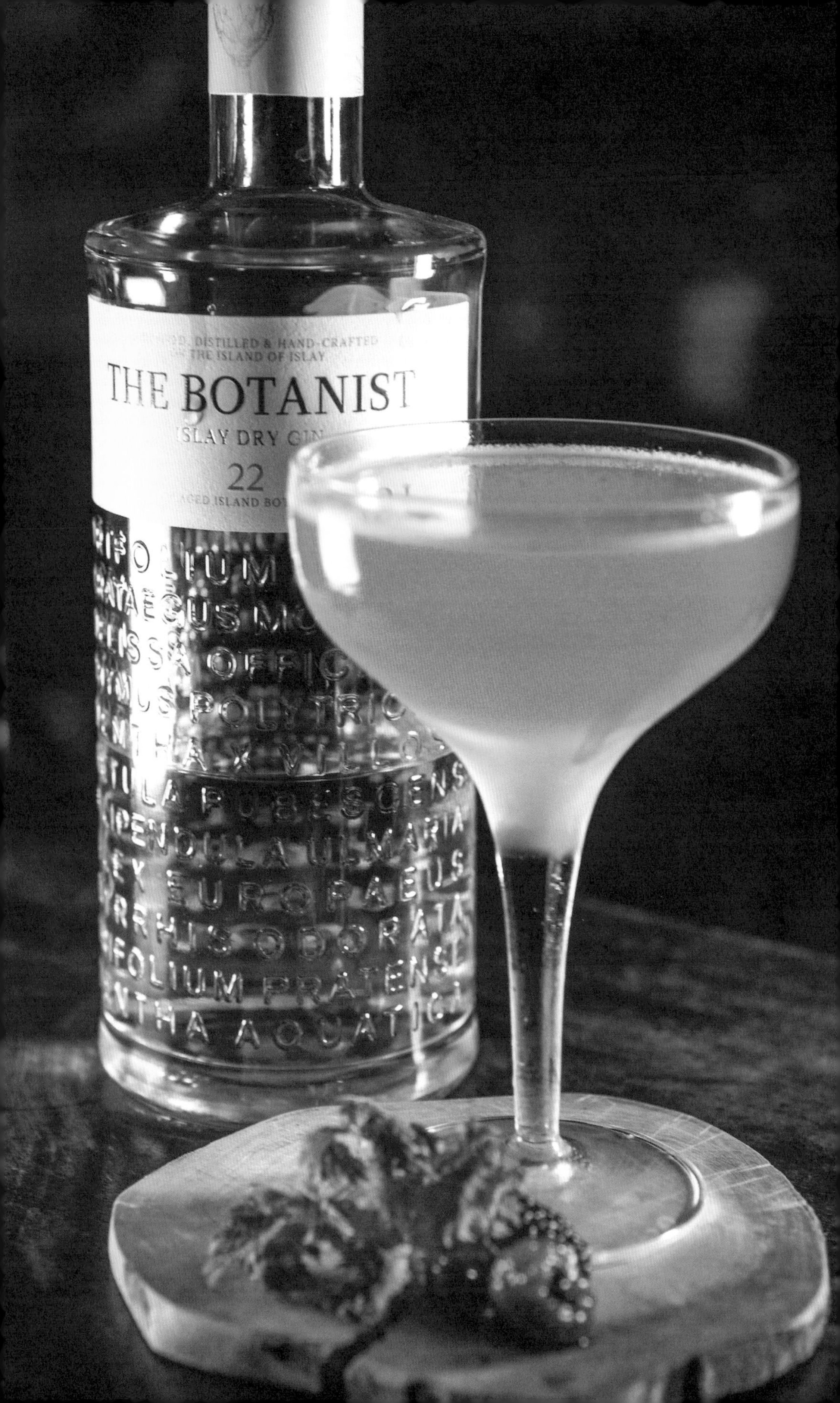
DISTILLED & HAND-CRAFTED
THE ISLAND OF ISLAY
THE BOTANIST
ISLAY DRY GIN
22

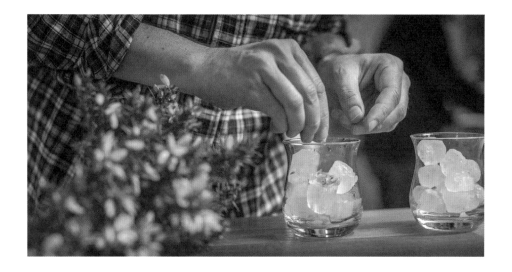

CREATIVE ADVERTISING

When the distillery was resurrected in 2004, there was no communications team or marketing team. Social media didn't exist in the same way; it didn't have a name. We had to be creative: distillery webcams, special bottlings, challenging convention. Our managing director wrote our blog articles and challenged the industry's press. We made noise about our production methods and our innovations. Some people loved it, and naturally some people loathed it. But it got people talking and Bruichladdich became the new kid on the block everyone was talking about.

As things have progressed, social media has become incredibly useful in delivering our messages and helping us reach out to a new and wider audience. For one thing, we have been able to connect with foragers, chefs, and bartenders all over the world and it is amazing to be a part of the conversation about gin and whisky online. From our humble beginnings, on a little island in the teeth of the Atlantic with dial-up internet, to our transition into a global brand, social media has been integral to our growth. But it needed the established and interesting conversations offline to take our dedicated followers online to continue shouting about us in a saturated market.

We have seen phenomenal growth in the popularity of The Botanist over the last few years. So much so, we are now the fastest-growing gin in the super-premium category and we now export to sixty-six countries. And as the popularity of gin continues to grow, with new distilleries and brands popping up on an almost daily basis, the category grows ever more competitive. If you are thinking of making your own gin, you have to believe in the brand, and we resolutely do.

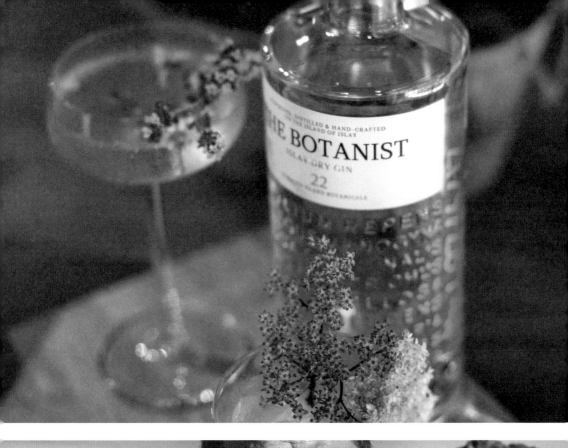
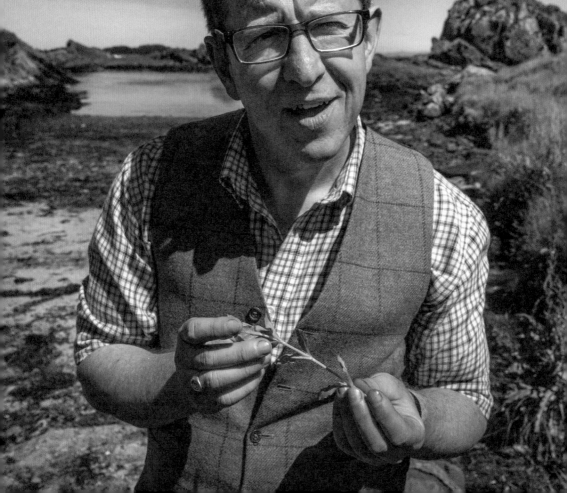

DISTILLING TO THE FUTURE

We are fortunate to have a global distribution network and The Botanist is sold all over the world. Having said that, one of our biggest sources of sales is our small distillery shop on Islay. Even though the distillery is owned by a larger brand, we have retained our independence. As far as possible, we do everything in-house on Islay. We believe it is important to keep employment on the island and give young people opportunities in the industry.

While retaining our independent spirit, but having a bigger company behind us, we have been able to break through the inevitable glass ceiling we would have reached without support. But when it comes to creativity, that is left to us. Remy bought us because of who we are and how we do things. That is why we sold to them: we now have the freedom to be creative but also the infrastructure to be able to do that. We have security to try new things and equally to be able to employ more people to make this happen.

"There is a pride in the workforce because this is a local product that is benefiting us all"

The distillery, much of it in part due to The Botanist, is now the biggest private employer on the island. This in turn means that more people are staying on the island, rather than moving to the mainland. The distillery is buzzing. There is a pride in the workforce because this is a local product that is benefiting us all.

With more funds at hand, Bruichladdich Distillery is currently exploring several renewable energy sources. These sustainable practices would complement the distillery's existing attempts to be more environmentally friendly, which currently includes reusing the hot waste water from distillation to run central heating. We also have two electric vehicles that are used to transport visitors to and from the distillery and by the staff team when hosting guests. We are determined to minimize the business's environmental impact and become 'completely green' in the future.

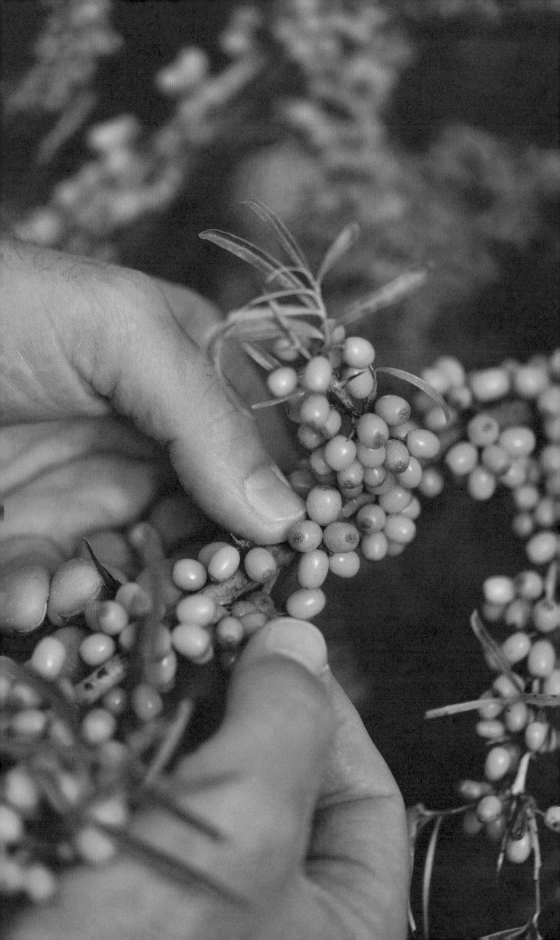

SEA
BUCKTHORN

Sea buckthorn is a shrub that produces edible berries that offer a variety of different tastes depending on when picked. Sought after by chefs as a luxury ingredient, the fruit can produce a fantastic, eye-catching colour. Sea buckthorn is considered to be a superfood as it is very high in vitamins and antioxidants. It is also a 'pioneer plant' and one of the first plants that started to grow after the end of the Ice Age 10,000 years ago.*

"One of the things that we love about growing our own berries is that we get to know all the different variations of them during the season"

Mads & Camilla Meisner, HØSTET

*Please note that sea buckthorn differs from buckthorn, which is in fact slightly poisonous.

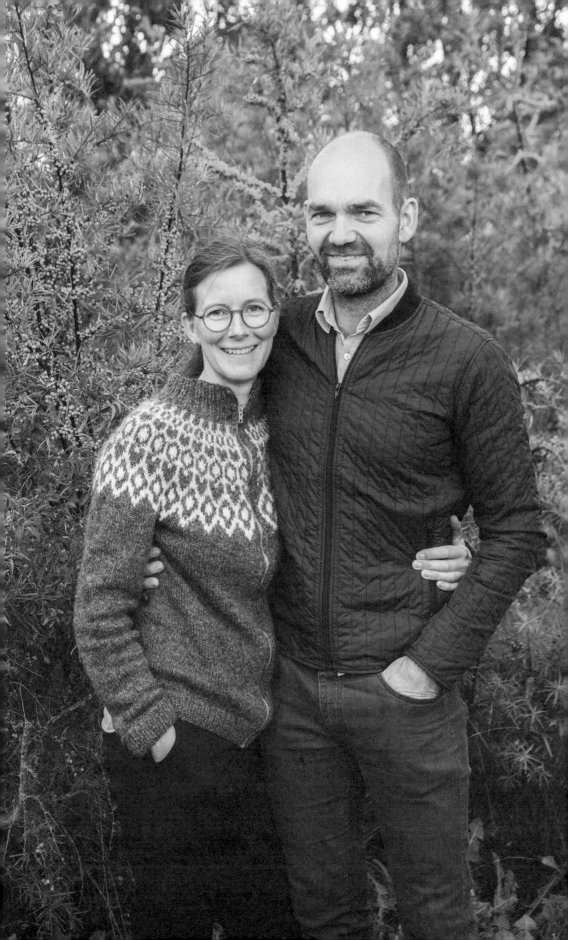

HØSTET

MADS & CAMILLA MEISNER

Bornholm, Denmark | hoestet.dk

After visiting the island of Bornholm in the summer of 2008 together with our kids, my husband and I came up with the idea of trying something new with our lives. Trying to create a less stressful life and living in the countryside on an island like Bornholm seemed very appealing.

At the same time, we read about a berry called sea buckthorn. We became very curious about these healthy berries and found a small sea buckthorn orchard in Sweden where we could sample them. We fell completely in love with the taste, which is a combination of orange, mango, and passionfruit – something very unusual compared to the other Nordic berries we knew.

Out of these experiences grew the idea of moving our family to Bornholm to start Denmark's first organic sea buckthorn orchard. Our name, 'HØSTET', means 'harvested' and we chose this name to represent our products because it says something about what is inside the jars and bottles. They are all produced with raw materials that have been gathered here on the unique island of Bornholm. We have been organically certified since 2013, before we harvested our first berries, as in Denmark it takes three years for fruit bushes to become certified organic.

GROWING A LIVELIHOOD

From the beginning, it has been Mads and me working on all the different parts of the business: establishing the orchard, harvesting, product development, labelling, selling, giving tours of the orchard, taking care of the farm shop, maintaining our online shop, and so on. We were both working in other areas before and this meant that from the start we were very much learning as we went along. Fortunately, Bornholm already had a pre-established culture of food start-ups – some new and some that have been operating for years – and this meant that there were experienced people whom we could ask for advice whenever we needed.

> "There are a lot of rules and legislation that must be followed; when you decide to do everything organic, there are even more"

When we started out, we established the first part of the orchard, with both of us working full-time in our existing jobs while we waited three years for the first berries to show. During these first three years we tended the orchard in our spare time. After harvesting the first small amount of berries, we decided that Mads should start to work full-time with the sea buckthorn as it is not just the harvesting and making that takes the time but also the business administration side of things. When you want to start a food-production business in Denmark (or anywhere, really), there are a lot of rules and legislation that must be followed; when you decide to do everything organic, there are even more. Going full-time allowed Mads to look into these issues and respond to them properly. A lot of reading was required and we asked people for advice and used advisors to help us understand everything we needed to. In Denmark, most legislation is available online so it is just a question of getting started and then making sure that you follow everything carefully.

After another six months, we decided that both of us needed to work full-time on developing the business, otherwise it would remain a part-time endeavour. This also meant that we needed to find a financial partner so that we could build an approved production kitchen on our farm and be able to pay a small salary to ourselves while still building the company.

As soon as we became a food start-up business on Bornholm, we worked an enormous number of hours in order to get things going. In the beginning, our kids thought that we were crazy to work so much because they couldn't really see the results of all the hard work. Now, several years later, they have become teenagers and both of them are working together with us to drive further success for our sea buckthorn business; it is a great joy to involve them in this work. We have good help from our kids, who have grown in the process, and also a few part-time workers. We are busy most of the year, but the first couple of months are quieter and this is when we make plans for the rest of the year.

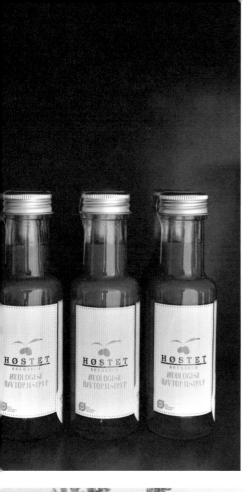
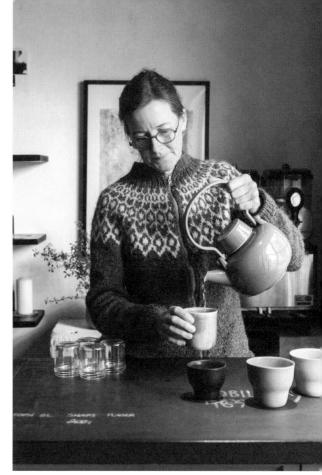
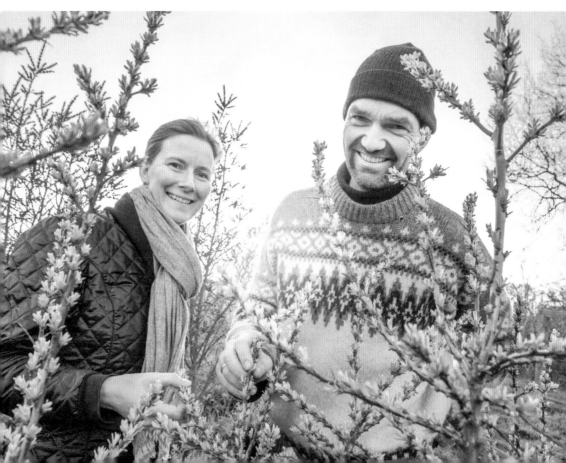

A MULTITUDE OF FLAVOUR

If you are passionate about an idea you have, there is a good chance that you think you will know what you are doing and how it will develop. But as time passes, things may work out very differently than you planned – as circumstances change, you become wiser, and your ideas develop.

When we started, we thought we were going to grow and harvest organic sea buckthorn berries and sell them to restaurants and producers around Denmark. We dreamed of showing this fantastic berry, with all its healthy content and great exotic taste, to everyone who had not come across it before. But eventually we learned that it would not be possible for us to build a sustainable business simply by growing and harvesting berries. We therefore became curious about what we could develop using the berries ourselves.

We started by making pure sea buckthorn marmalade. It turned out that not very many people had tasted this wonderful food stuff in its pure form; it is often mixed with other fruits because it is an expensive berry that can be difficult to find. Shortly after we cooked our first batch of marmalade, we won first prize in a competition judged by some of Denmark's best chefs. This gave us a lot of encouragement.

We have since developed a small range of sea buckthorn products alongside the marmalade, and all of them offer different varieties of the sea buckthorn taste. For example: when you taste our marmalade you get a creamy, intense, and exotic taste; when you taste our hundred per cent sea buckthorn juice you get the very sour and pure flavour of the berries; if you taste the syrup, the flavour is more caramelized, but still has a hint of acidity; our dried flakes do not have an intense taste, but offer a beautiful colour and a fine hint of the fruit's flavour. This exploration and showcasing of sea buckthorn has been a key issue for us from the beginning. We want to highlight the sea buckthorn flavour in different varieties, but always as pure as possible and with as few ingredients as possible.

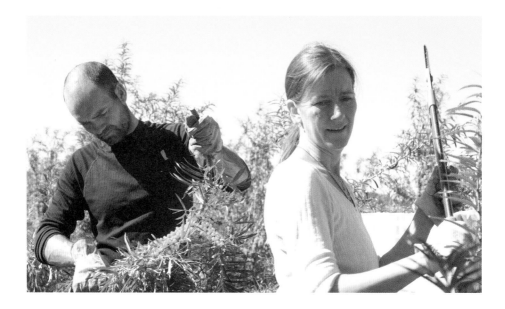

One of the things that we love about growing our own berries is that we get to know all the different variations of them during the season. It means that we can taste the berries, not only when they are ripe and orange, but also when they are green and unripe. This sometimes creates ideas for new products and possibilities for how we can use the fruit in different ways. We taste the berries once or twice a week all the way through the season and this gives us a better idea about when to harvest both the unripe and the ripe berries. This also makes it possible for us to explain the taste of the berries when someone asks us about it. The unripe berries do not have the familiar exotic taste, but they have a fine acidity reminiscent of gooseberry. Chefs we work with love that they now have a 'new' berry to experiment with. We want to share our excitement for this delicacy, and the better we get to know the berry and leaves, the more opportunities for their use we find. It would be very sad if these things were kept a secret.

TASTE FROM WASTE

As we started harvesting the berries and learned how difficult and time-consuming it was, it became very important for us to use up every single part of the raw materials. Out of this need came several products that we would most probably not have developed if we did not grow and harvest the berries ourselves. We use up everything, from the juice of the berries, to the skin, the nut inside, and also the leaves. Nothing is wasted. During dry summers we also collect water from the process of washing the berries and use it to water the new plants in the orchard. All plastic used in our production is collected and sent for recycling. There are still lots of things that we would like to work with in regards to sustainability, but we try to improve and adjust wherever it is possible

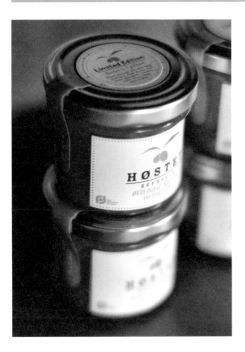 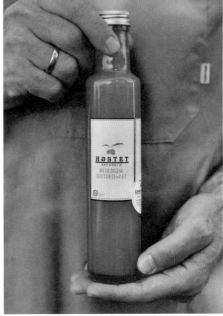

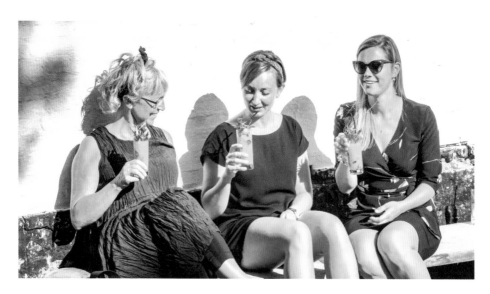

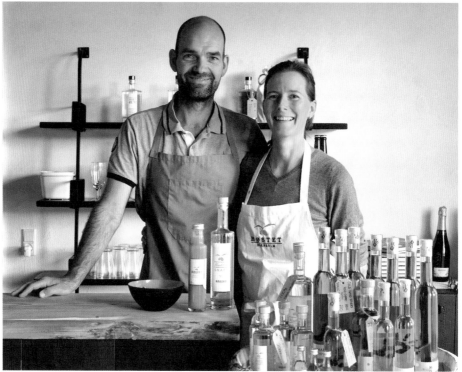

SUNSHINE ON GLASS

We use glass for most of our packing. Not only is it necessary for food safety in our production processes, it is also a recyclable material and it beautifully displays the wonderful colour of sea buckthorn. This colour has become part of our story. We call it 'sunshine on glass', and together with the name 'HØSTET' it conveys a lot about our products.

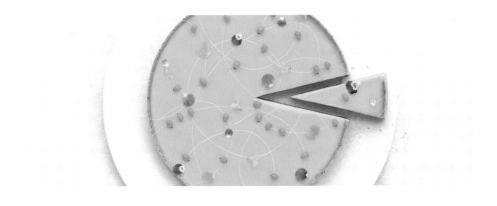

SHARING A STORY

We have always experienced huge interest in the fact that our process is *jord til bord* – soil to table. By this we mean that we grow the produce and take care of the whole process right up until it reaches the homes of our customers. There is an increasing interest from people about understanding where their food is coming from and how it has been produced. The people we meet like to learn more about their food and visit us because we know something about sea buckthorn, its use, and its high nutrient values.

Bornholm is a holiday island and every year we experience an increase in the number of visitors to our farm shop. From the beginning, we learned that people like to experience everything. They would like a tour around the orchard; they are interested to hear both our story about moving to Bornholm and the story about the berries; then they would like to taste the different products. Luckily, most people also buy lots of products to take home for friends and themselves. This creates a very genuine experience for them that helps to sell the authenticity of our product. We try to give everyone the same attention, because we believe that everyone who visits us, tastes our products, and hears our story is a potential ambassador for HØSTET.

Most people also find that our products are very honest because they contain few ingredients and are prepared in an artisanal way. This works very well with sharing our story on social media because sea buckthorn looks beautiful in pictures, as does our orchard, the view over the Baltic Sea, the marmalade on a biscuit, or when we are filling the jars by hand. Our farm shop looks better than a supermarket and the drinks that we make during the summer look delicious. For a smaller business like ours, social media is an effective way to show what we are working with.

We sell approximately fifty per cent through our resellers and fifty per cent from our farm shop and food markets. We have decided not to work with distributors because we like to have direct contact with our customers. Our products are special and high-end. It is therefore important to us that whoever sells our products also knows our story and can tell customers how they are made. Our farm shop obviously brings in revenue but it can also work as a test shop for new products. We can test them during the summer when we have plenty of visitors, and then take the product all the way to our resellers later if we decide to. If we only sell a product from our farm shop, there is less legislation to follow.

'JORD TIL BORD'

Orchards Every year we try to expand the orchard a little bit more. We do this by digging up the new root sprouts from the old orchard, and adding them to the new orchard. We tend the orchard all months of the year, some more than others, but as far as the weather allows we have work to do there all year round.

Harvesting Depending on the summer, we start harvesting in the beginning or middle of August. We cut the branches and take them directly to the freezing house where they are kept frozen until we can start shaking the berries and leaves from the branches. We feel very fortunate that we have created a job for ourselves in which we also get to do the actual harvesting, because that is something very special.

Shaken not stirred When the branches have been frozen for four to five days, we can start the process of shaking the berries and leaves from the branches. While we do this, everything is still frozen and kept that way until we start the sorting of the berries from the leaves.

Sorting Before we can start to use the berries for the production, we need to sort them from the leaves. We have a special machine that helps us with this, but it is still a time-consuming process. Here the berries and leaves remain frozen and go back in the freezer after sorting.

Washing Before we start production, the berries must be washed. We take them out to defrost and then shower them carefully in small amounts. At this stage we also carry out a final sorting of the berries.

Making Now production can start. We have developed all our products ourselves, and everything is cooked or dried in our kitchen on our farm.

Selling From April to October we open our farm shop, which is located right next to the orchard. We are open for everyone a couple of hours every afternoon. We then we receive bigger groups of guests, who have pre-booked a tour around the orchard followed by a tasting in the farm shop.

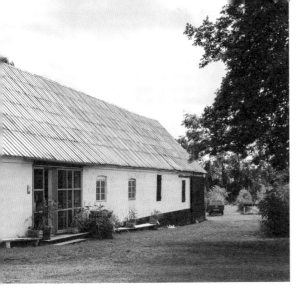

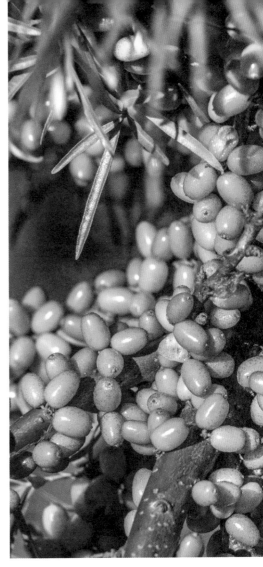

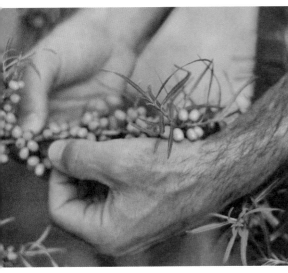

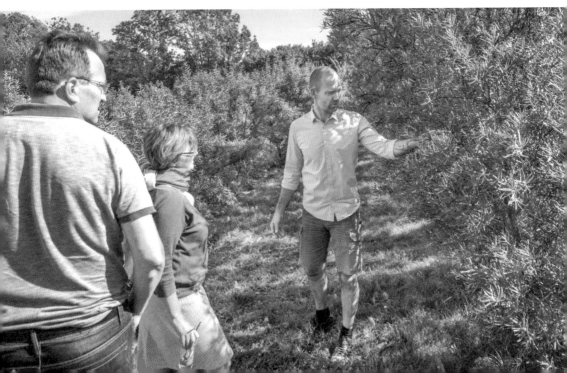

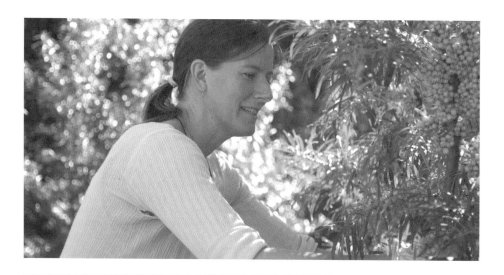

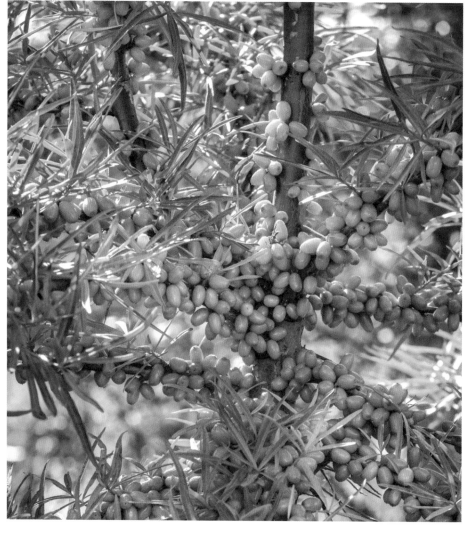

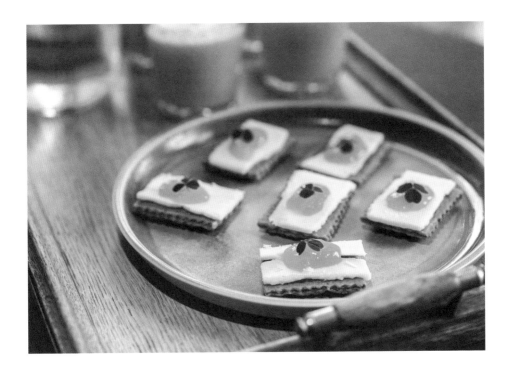

MAINTAINING AUTHENTICITY

Our marmalade is cooked in small batches for a short time, which makes it possible for us to keep the beautiful bright colour and fresh taste of sea buckthorn. This is a key issue for our production and one of the things that we will never change. The harvest of sea buckthorn must take place at the right time in addition to when the berries are ripe. The berries are rich in omega 3, 6, 7, and 9, and this means that when we harvest they must be frozen shortly after the branches have been cut, to ensure the oil in the juice is kept fresh. We have met people that thought they did not like sea buckthorn, but this is often because it does not take many rancid berries to contaminate a whole batch. We protect the processes that have an effect on the quality of our products; however, we optimize on the techniques that can affect income and expenditure. The cooking will stay the same, but we could optimize, for example, the date stamping, labelling, maybe the washing and sorting of the berries and leaves, without it having an adverse effect on the taste and quality of our products.

Since storytelling is a big part of our strategy, it is also important for us to stay true to our story, which means that our production should not become industrialized. In regards to our kind of production, I think that we would have crossed the line into industrialization if we did not come in contact with the berries during the production. But we taste the berries before, during, and after harvest; we also sort the berries, wash them, and press them. It is difficult to define the exact size that is ideal for our business, both in regard to employees and turnover, but being conscious about it is the best we can do.

THE FUTURE

We love the fact that we are now working together with our children in the company that we have started, but we do not expect them to stay here for good, at least not until they have left the island and experienced a bigger part of the world. And who knows, maybe they will end up back here on Bornholm, older and wiser, and find that life in the countryside is lovely. Until then, we are enjoying the fact that we are experiencing increased demand for local food. For the first time in decades, Bornholm is experiencing an increase in its population. Among them are young people, who want to grow vegetables, create a food-start-up, or just be closer to nature.

We definitely hope to be able to share all our knowledge on sea buckthorn – both growing it and processing it. One way to do that could be that instead of developing our company into a huge sea buckthorn factory, we aim to create a meaningful and sustainable workplace for the people we employ and ourselves. We would like to grow our business to a size that fits our environment and our farm and then start to use some of our time on coaching other people who want to start similar projects, either here in Denmark or abroad. We want to take care of nature and its resources, both for our own and our children's sake. We try to implement sustainability in our way of living and our way of working – for example, we have solar panels on our roof and all plastic used in our production is collected and sent for recycling. There are many other things that we would like to introduce in regards to sustainability, so we try to improve and adjust wherever it is possible.

> "What we love most about the new life that we have created for ourselves is that we have the opportunity to share our passion with so many interesting people"

Denmark is very strict on how you may claim food to be healthy. Therefore, when it comes to marketing our products, so far we have focused on the taste and the use of pure organic raw materials rather than their direct health benefits. It seems like a no-brainer to focus on the nutritional advantages with such a healthy berry as sea buckthorn though, so this is an opportunity that we would like to explore a lot more in the future. For now, being a small business still in the phase of establishing our company, we are trying to find the balance between developing new products and the daily running of the company. If you are a creative person, it will never be a problem to come up with new ideas. The challenge will always be to try to make your ideas sustainable and reach black numbers on the bottom line.

What we love most about the new life that we have created for ourselves is that we have the opportunity to share our passion with so many interesting people. We do not work with the same tasks all year round, but divide our time between lots of different things. And without knowing it, when we fell in love with sea buckthorn it turned out to be a berry with so many different possibilities.

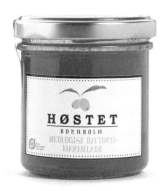

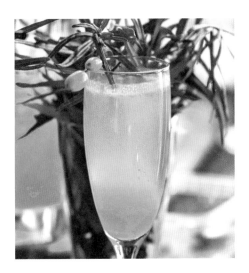

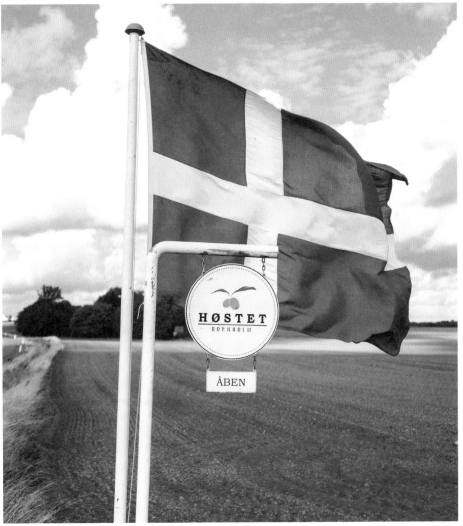

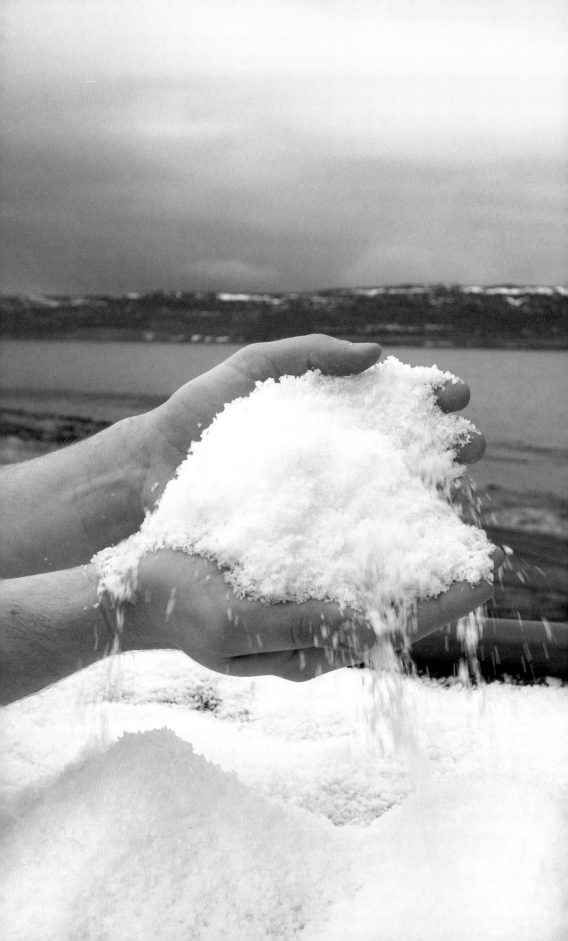

SALT

Throughout history, salt has had a significant value and currency indicative of its importance as a food seasoning and a preservative. Sea salt is one of the most natural forms of edible salt as it can be found in vast quantities in the oceans. Unlike table salt, it is extracted simply by evaporating the seawater, so it is more eco-friendly than other salt production methods and not hugely processed. The production methods of sea salt as opposed to table salt also mean that its natural benefits are retained. Laden with minerals essential to our health, sea salt is reputed to be beneficial to electrolyte balance, blood pressure, and muscle cramps, and can also be put to good use as a balancing or cleansing ingredient in skin-friendly beauty products.

"We have a personal connection to our product, so we will always hand-harvest the salt... This experience could never be replaced by equipment or technology"

Björn Steinar Jónsson, Saltverk

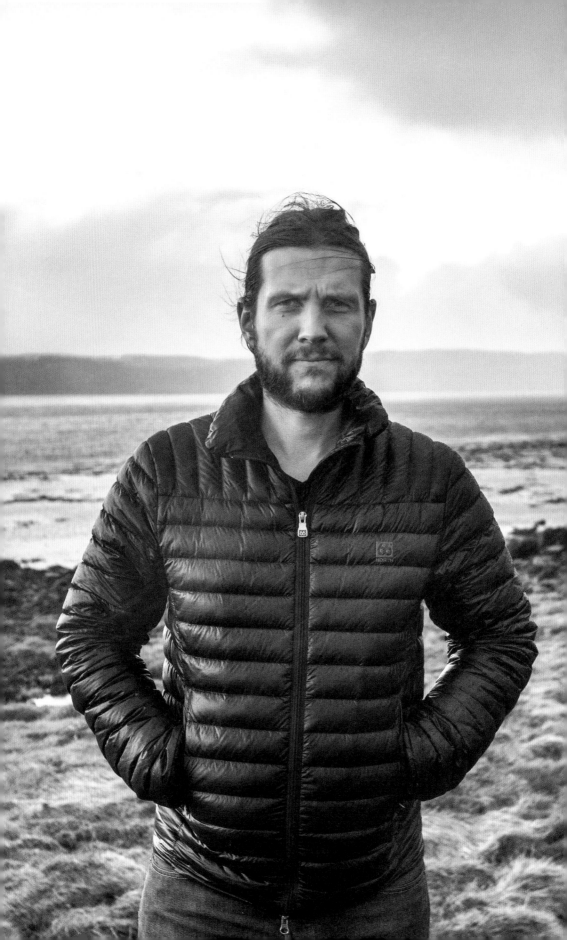

SALTVERK

BJÖRN STEINAR JÓNSSON

Reykjanes, Iceland | saltverk.com

Saltverk tells a story of sustainable produce, crafted in a remote location, and of how to be transparent and sustainable in everything you do as a food producer. We are one of the few entirely sustainable sea salt producers in the world, using geothermal energy to evaporate seawater. The sea salt flakes left behind from this process are handmade, pyramid-like crystal structures that contain the flavour and taste of the Nordic region from which the raw materials used in it are derived. Saltverk sea salt includes minerals necessary for the human body and embodies a calmness reminiscent of the location of its tranquil production surroundings. It is used in many of the best restaurants and in the homes of food enthusiasts around the world.

FOLLOWING A PASSION

The idea for Saltverk germinated while I was living in Copenhagen for ten years studying to become an engineer. As a self-described 'foodie', I had a deep interest in food and restaurants, and at the time there was a lot going on surrounding food in Copenhagen. During these years (specifically 2008–2010) new foods were emerging, a lot of restaurants were popping up, and international chefs flocked to the city. My interest and knowledge of production and manufacturing methods combined with a fascination with food to create the idea and drive behind Saltverk.

I am originally from Iceland, but after the financial crisis in Iceland at that time, if I wanted to go back home and needed a job, I had to create it myself. There weren't many jobs available at the time, and certainly not any with a more international perspective. Iceland has a lot of renewable resources and opportunities to harness geothermal energy, but they were mainly being used by large international companies in ways that were not very sustainable. There has been a lot of debate about how these natural resources should be used. I wanted to take advantage of the renewable energy source in Iceland in a way that would be completely sustainable, to create an honest and eco-friendly product. It is a small island and no one was producing salt in Iceland at that time, so I started to experiment with adapting salt production methods that harness geothermal energy, and Saltverk evolved from there.

> "It feels like a real privilege to be able to make something for some of the world's best restaurants. It gives me contact with interesting people every day and the chance to work collaboratively with other businesses"

Before I came back to Iceland and started Saltverk, I worked for an IT company with 400,000 employees. Going from that busy environment to setting up a salt manufacturing business alone was therefore a huge shift. Previously working as one of many, I had felt alienated and like I didn't fit in a large organization. Having the chance to make something for people that they could use and enjoy, and being able to deliver it directly to customers, was extremely fulfilling and rewarding, and continues to be so. There is a feeling of self-sufficiency in being able to make a product and deliver it to a customer and see it being used. It feels like a real privilege to be able to make something for some of the world's best restaurants. It gives me contact with interesting people every day and the chance to work collaboratively with other businesses.

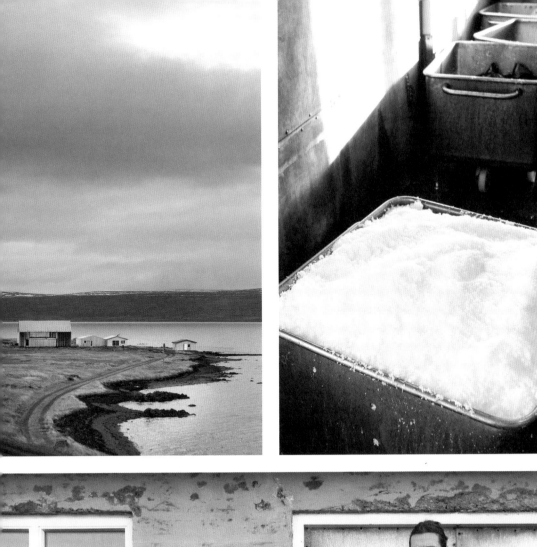
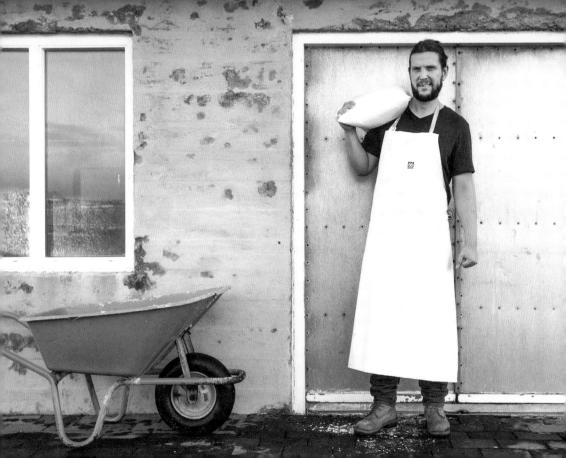

HARVESTING SALT

When I started Saltverk, as far as I knew, no one in the world was using geothermal energy to produce salt. Sea salt used to be produced in this way in the Westfjords region of Iceland around 250 years ago, but it sadly came to an end. In 2011, however, we looked back to these methods and considered how we could adapt them to be used today.

Seawater is the raw material used for making sea salt and is around three per cent salinity; we need to extract ninety per cent of the water in order to create the sea salt flakes. The main step of the process is evaporating the liquid, leaving just the flaky salt. We use the geyser water from the hot springs of Reykjanes in the preheating, boiling, and drying process for our salt. This geothermal energy is the sole energy source used, which means that during our whole process we have zero carbon footprint on the environment and have no carbon dioxide or methane emissions.

> The seawater is pumped into open pans using electric pumps at the bottom of the fjord, with the electricity coming from local hydropower plants. We preheat the seawater in the pans until it becomes a strong brine, with a salinity level of seventeen to twenty per cent.

⬇

> The brine is boiled until white crystals appear on the surface and slowly fall to the bottom of the pan.

⬇

> The salt is drawn across the pan and any remaining liquid is drained.

⬇

> The salt flakes are then dried and packaged for our customers.

We have a personal connection to our product, so we will always hand-harvest the salt. Everyone who works for the company starts out by going to the factory and harvesting salt. We train our salt makers to control the quality of the salt, and they develop an experienced eye for the perfect product. This is a very important element of the manufacturing process because our consumers include many of the world's best chefs, who demand a high-quality product. This experience could never be replaced by equipment or technology.

I believe it is a good thing that we have brought salt production back to Iceland once more. It makes the most of the natural resources around us in an eco-friendly way. For this reason, and to keep a national heritage alive, it is very important to pass on our salt production methods; I hope that Iceland will be able to continue producing sea salt using geothermal energy for future generations to come.

A BENEVOLENT ENVIRONMENT

Reykjanes, where the North Arctic Ocean stream goes down the bay of Ísafjarðardjúp, has some of the cleanest seawater imaginable. It is home to a lively range of wildlife, including whales, seals, and birds. The area is also home to a number of active geysers, from which the place derives its name.

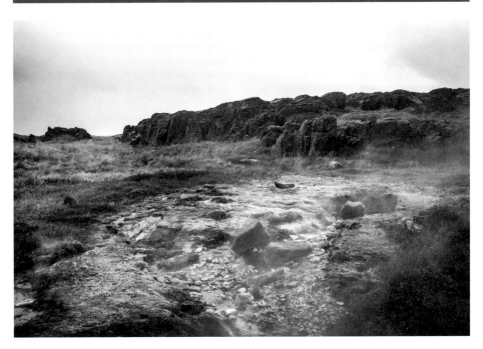

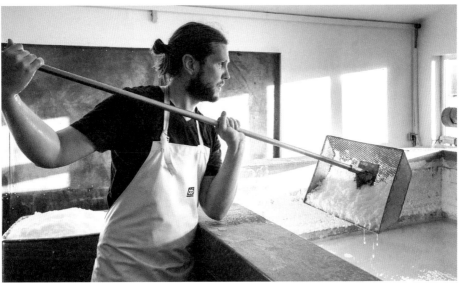

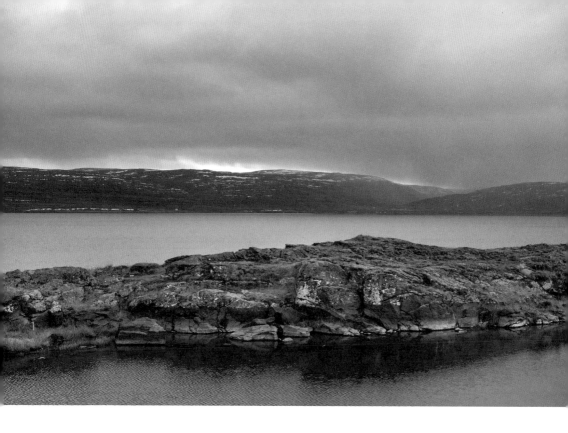

MAINTAINING INTEGRITY

As you can see, our process is very honest – we are just evaporating seawater and not adding anything to the product. We are simply harnessing sustainable resources to contribute to a more sustainable world. We strive to retain this honesty and transparency throughout the rest of our business, and we do this in a number of ways.

- We try to **work with environmentally friendly companies** where possible, working with other sustainable or eco-conscious businesses in the areas in which our product is sold, in order to become part of the sustainable ecosystem.

- In terms of production, we leave **zero impact** on the environment.

- We **offset our carbon footprint** by planting trees through a charity called Kolvidur, which was founded by the Icelandic Forestry Association and the Icelandic Environment Association.

- We only transport our product for **export by sea**, instead of air, as ships produce much less carbon dioxide.

- We use **glass instead of plastic** for our packaging and the paper we use on this comes from **renewable Nordic sources**.

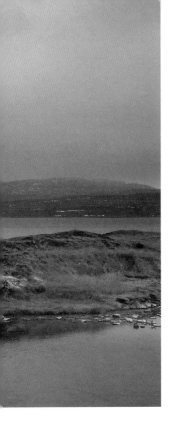

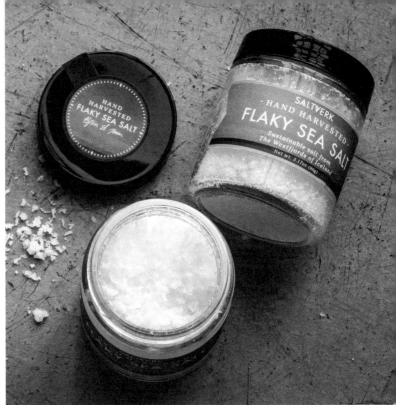

As industries become more sustainable and innovative, and more environmentally friendly packaging solutions are developed, we will be able to take advantage of them even further. We are always looking to improve and grow – for example, we are currently developing refillable and reusable packaging to be used in restaurants.

From a legal point of view, all of our products need to be approved by the local food authority and checked for the correct health and safety regulations for food manufacturing. We also need to follow regulations for selling food in the United States and Europe. However, as we set ourselves higher standards than what is required, regulations are easy to adhere to. Some of our customers also demand more information and certification for certain requirements, which we are always happy to supply. We want to align the product with our own values as consumers who want to buy sustainably manufactured products.

PERSON-TO-PERSON CONNECTION

We made the decision to work directly with all the markets that we operate in. We have used distributors in the past but we prefer to market our product ourselves because we feel we are the best people to market it. We do work with some partners, in small aspects of the business, but focus on having a direct connection to the customers ourselves.

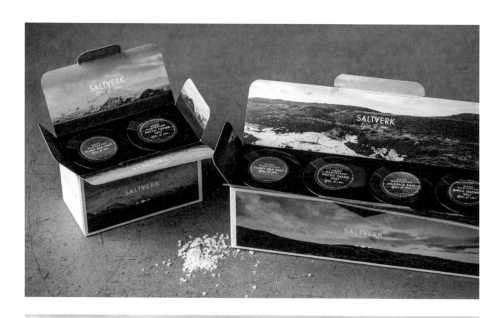

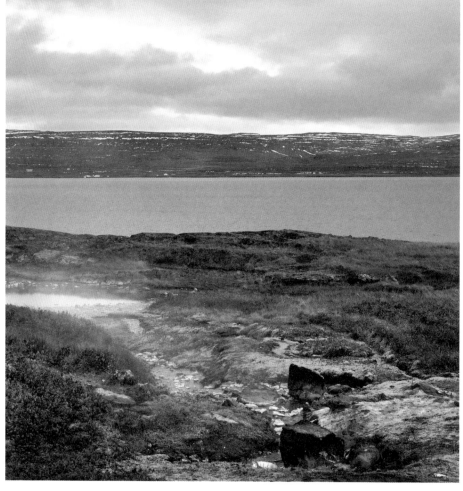

SUSTAINING OURSELVES

We have had many battles to get to where we are today – it hasn't been a fairy-tale experience and there are many potential threats to the business that still exist. For example, as we operate our business in the north of Iceland, the increased effects of global warming could have a huge impact on our production. In Iceland, we also experience volcanic eruptions and a major eruption can disturb production.

"We are conscious that we are catering to a more considerate generation, who want to pay for higher quality, transparency, and sustainability"

One of the biggest threats to Saltverk, however, is the consumer environment – if attitudes change and the consumer industry doesn't continue to become more sustainable and transparent, then we could see damaging effects to our growth and marketability. I think there has been a major shift in food production for the better, and hopefully it will continue to move in this direction. Just before Saltverk was launched in 2011, eco-consciousness and integrity had become an important, ever-increasing trend. What we are starting to see is the appreciation of the sustainability aspect of our work. We are conscious that we are catering to a more considerate generation, who want to pay for higher quality, transparency, and sustainability. Since the beginning, we have been very transparent in what we do; anyone can visit us and see how we make our product. This is something you see more and more of, especially in food and drink. I think previous generations were more focused on mass-production and people became disconnected from the food that was on their plates.

Large organizations often don't want to show the consumer what they are doing, but today's consumer wants to know and have traceability of their food, all the way back to the origins of the product. It can be seen in many aspects of food production, for example with restaurants and other food producers we work with. Every stage of the supply chain is functioning in a sustainable manner. Other sustainable food producers make a conscious decision to use our handcrafted salt because it aligns with their own vision. This is very much where we fit as a producer.

APPRECIATING YOUR CRAFT

If you are thinking about starting your own artisan food business, make sure it is something that you appreciate – the craft and work that needs to be done, from manufacturing to distributing and selling of the product. Design your business in a way that suits you and your lifestyle. Consider whether you are ready for it – you can very much become a slave to your own company as you can to someone else's company! You need to understand what it may entail before you start and ensure that you will get joy from it.

GROWTH

When I first started Saltverk, I was very much involved in harvesting, packaging, and delivering the salt. As we have grown, my role has changed, and I now act as the ambassador and sales representative of the business. I have also taken on a management role to organize the smooth running of the business, as well as being the main point of contact for our biggest customers across the markets that we work in.

We sell our product in the home market in Iceland, as well as the international export market – mainly the United States and Scandinavia. Our salt can be found in high-end food stores and also used by restaurants and other food producers. We mainly sell directly to customers and producers and our products can be bought off the shelves in food stores and supermarkets, so they are accessible to the everyday consumer. We do have a lot of competition, but it motivates us to improve and grow our business and product. We aim to create a mutually successful product for our stockists and ourselves.

"I work to constantly grow the company in a sustainable way"

We will never be a large-scale industrial operation, but we live in a modern world and there are some areas where we can use technology to our advantage, such as during the packaging process. Similarly, 250 years ago stainless steel wasn't available, but it is incredibly useful so today it is a crucial element of the production method. Working as a food producer in the twenty-first century means we have to adapt our methods to suit today's food industry standards, which has been a rewarding challenge. I work to constantly grow the company in a sustainable way.

Our method is an adaptation of the traditional method of creating sea salt flakes with the aim of producing them in a more sustainable and resourceful way. We gather salt throughout the year and have scaled up every year since we began. We sell everything that we are able to create. We will never change the handcrafted elements of our business. This limits how much we can produce but means we maintain ourselves as an honest and sustainable producer.

STANDING OUT FROM THE CROWD

When you have a product on the shelf, it is competing with many other products, so it needs to be able to speak for itself and deliver a message – what it is, where it comes from, how it is made. That's a very difficult task. We started working with a design company in Copenhagen in 2014, which really succeeded in communicating the message that we wanted to convey through our branding. We changed the packaging from a previous design that was good but didn't communicate enough about our company. As a result of this change, our packaging plays an important role in getting our products from the shelves into the hands of the consumers.

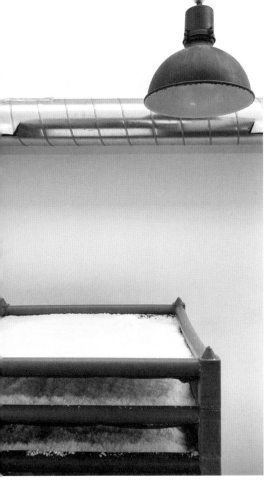

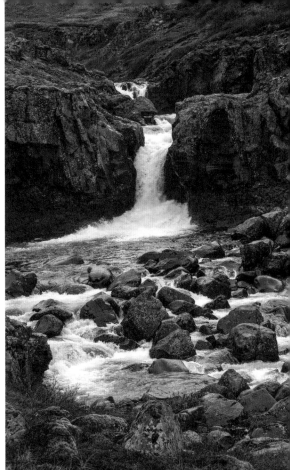

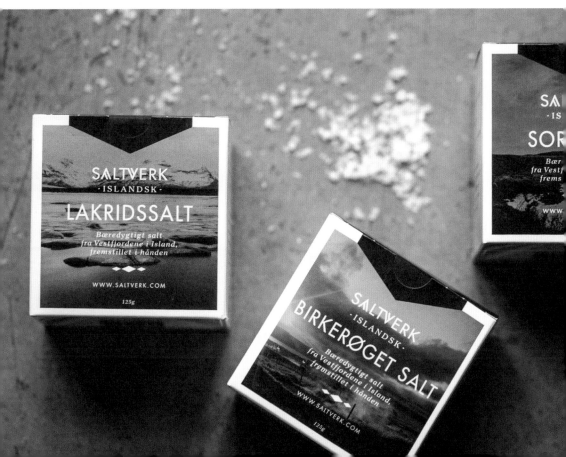

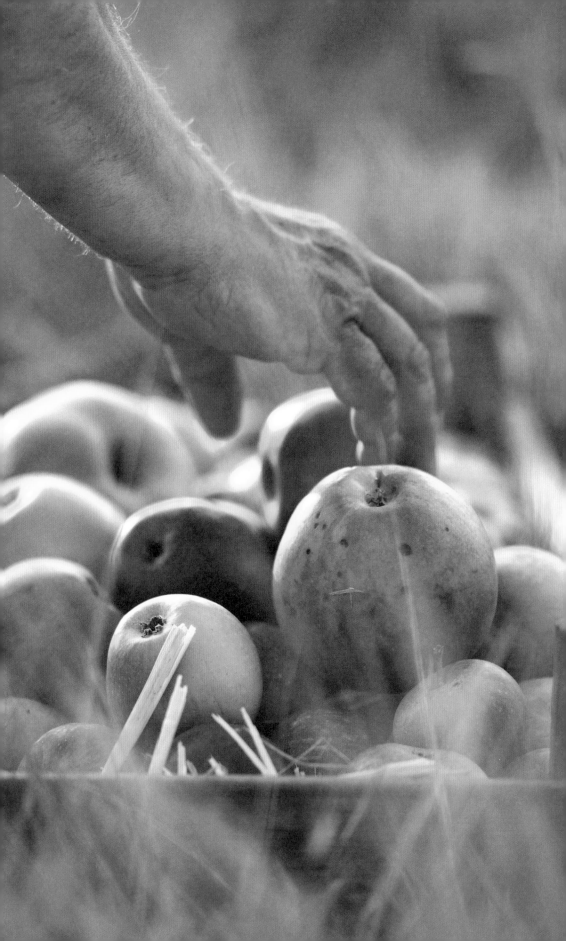

HEIRLOOM FRUITS

Heirloom fruits come from heritage plants that have often been passed down from generation to generation. They have many benefits for our own health and for the health of our planet. They have had time to adapt themselves perfectly to their local environment, negating the need for harmful pesticides, and their variety and diversity promotes larger-scale biodiversity and a healthier ecosystem.

As well as being nutritious and tasting great, heirloom fruits bring with them their own cultural and historical significance. Forced into the margins by high-yielding and supermarket-friendly sweet, 'perfect-looking' fruit, heirloom fruits are experiencing a revival as discerning consumers support sustainable, small-scale growers. By choosing to cultivate and to eat heirloom fruits, we are not only choosing healthy alternatives to mass-produced commodities, we are also ensuring that these diverse plants are protected for the future.

"It inspires me to think that some of
the apple varieties I have planted go
back to the fourteenth century"

David De Vleeschauwer, Verger Du Nord

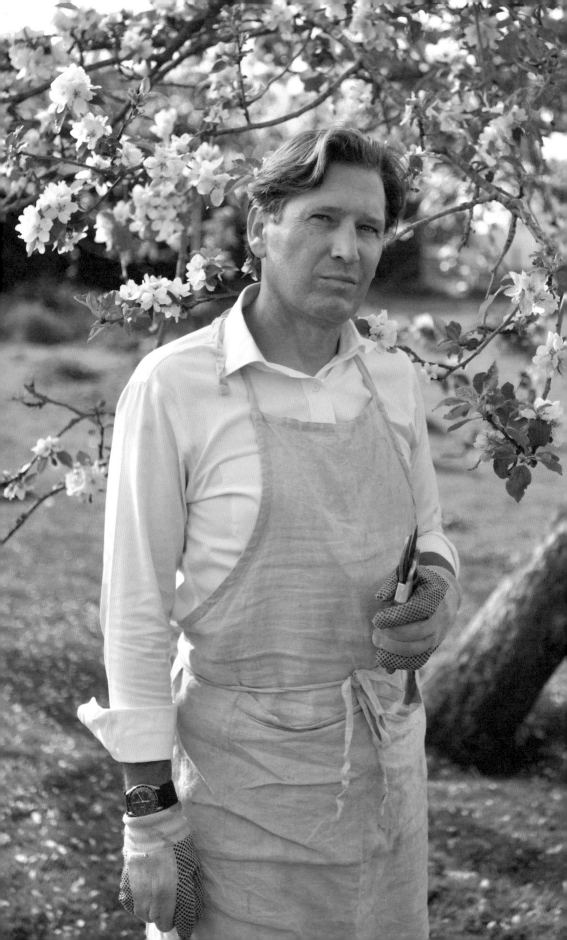

VERGER DU NORD

DAVID DE VLEESCHAUWER

Watou, Belgium & Steenvoorde, France | instagram.com/vergerdunord

---

A few years ago, I started restoring the old orchards located next to the homestead of my historic hops farm. The name Verger du Nord (Orchard of the North) originated from the fact that the farm is located almost on the border between Belgium and northern France. As a photographer I travel the world constantly and I started noticing the urge and drive from people in different countries and locations to go back to basics and preserve traditions and heritage. I started doing some research and bought a very extensive collection of old variety and local high-stem fruit trees to give the old orchard a second life. In the last couple of years a total of 200 historic varieties have been planted in the old orchards in Belgium and France. With every planting session, my knowledge and fascination grew and my drive to save old apple varieties increased.

The apples are now used to make juices and ciders, which are then used by chefs we collaborate with. We hand-pick the apples, take them to the presser, and try to obtain a juice that stands out and is purer in taste than anything else available on the market. I am proud to give my family's farm a second life and a new purpose, but there is also a joy in knowing that I am saving an agricultural heritage in Belgium. The high-stem fruit trees I plant are mainly from Belgium and northern France, or originate from neighbouring countries, and were widely popular and planted in the old days.

A SENSE OF HISTORY

Since ancient times in Europe, there have been increases and decreases in preference for certain types of fruit growing. For example, high-stem orchards peaked during the eighteenth and nineteenth centuries, whereas after the Second World War, mainly due to the availability of pesticides and the fear of famine, low-stem fruit tree orchards replaced high-stem orchards. European governments handed out subsidies to destroy these 'inferior' high-stem fruit-tree orchards and to replace them with the more productive low-stem varieties. All this led to an organized eradication of many historical and local fruit varieties.

In the space of a few years, a region's agricultural landscape could be thoroughly turned upside down. As an example, after the introduction of the train as an efficient means of transport, more than ninety per cent of the 85,000 hectares of orchards in Belgium disappeared, and with them also fruit heritage and related customs. Fortunately, as a counter-reaction, associations like the Belgian Nationale Boomgaard Stichting (National Orchard Foundation) popped-up in the 1970s. A collection of 500 fruit varieties was quickly established and the current gene bank now has 300 varieties of apples, pears, cherries, plums, and other fruit varieties from local, national, and international origins.

It inspires me to think that some of the apple varieties I have planted go back to the fourteenth century and I enjoy learning about how fruit varieties came to life and who created them. Sometimes apple or pear varieties refer to their creator or family members, like the Louise-Bonne d'Avranches, created by a Frenchman in 1770 for his dear wife called Louise de Longueval. The Reine des Reinettes (or the King of the Peppins) dates back to 1700 and is a sour apple preferably picked at the end of summer or early autumn, and which can last the whole winter. Going through the hundreds of apple and pear varieties is like reading a history book about gardens and orchards planted centuries ago. Some of these varieties are still here but many of them are almost extinct or no longer grown and sold in the shops. Thankfully, I have noticed a movement of the public towards more locally sourced and traceable food.

A MYRIAD OF VARIETIES

Choosing which varieties to grow is extremely interesting once you know the background and what the fruit was used for in the past. I recently discovered an old variety of pear called Smoutpeer (butter pear) dating back to 1396, perfect for making a chunky pear sauce and preserving it. Cabaret or President Van Dievoet is an apple that was created in 1878. It is only harvested in October and only after three months of resting in a cold, dark place is the fruit ready to eat. Reinet Bakker Parmentier from Kortrijk (a city in West Flanders) was used in the past specifically for apple pie. Plovine pears are used mainly in preserves and are not eaten raw. These are just a few examples.

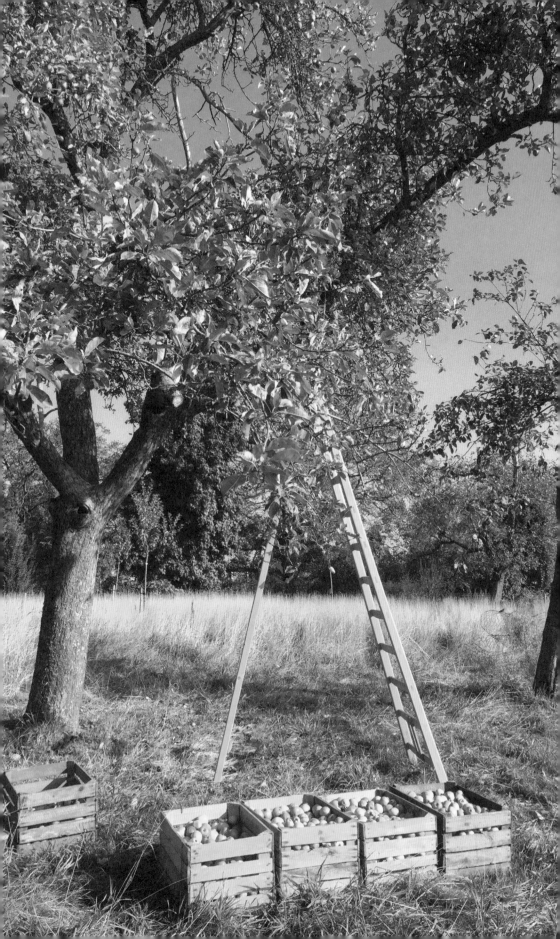

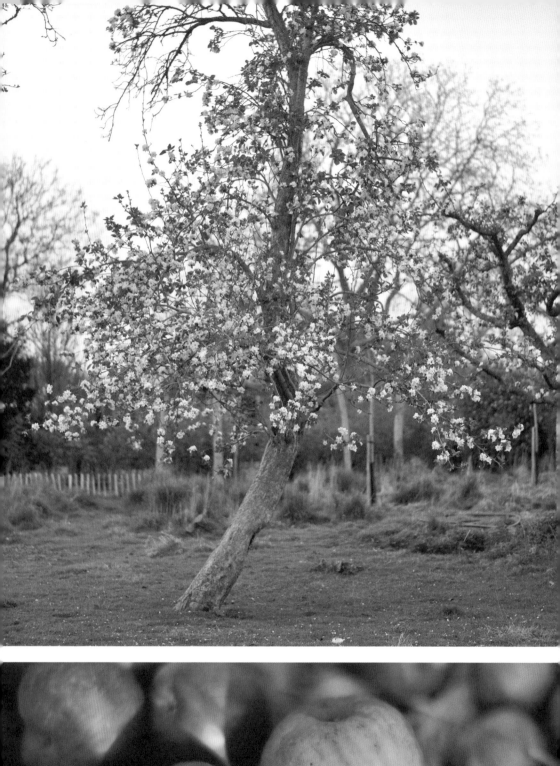
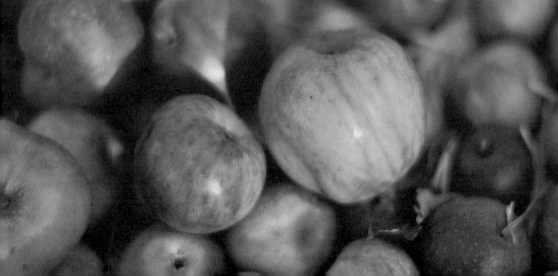

THE BENEFITS OF SMALL-SCALE, LOCAL GROWING

A key element of the project for me is bringing more awareness to a wider audience about the existence of old apple and pear varieties with local roots. When the consumer is more aware of what they are eating or drinking, their taste buds also develop. All of a sudden somebody will taste a huge difference between industrially produced apple juice, syrupy sweet and sticky with plenty of added sugar and water, and our cloudy, unfiltered, tangy apple juice.

Nowadays, the varieties of fruit people buy in the supermarket are narrowed down to just a small fraction of all existing varieties. Fruit bred for sweetness might appeal most to consumers in the supermarket, but modern de-bittered fruits tend to contain less of the phytonutrients that give fruits and vegetables many of their protective health benefits. Heirloom fruits offer better taste and better nutrition.

We think carefully about where we plant the trees as pollination is vital to create an almost self-sufficient ecosystem where trees, insects, birds, small mammals, cows, and sheep interact. Next to the orchard I have begun planting over 150 varieties of herbs, which help with the biodiversity of the farm. We also started introducing chickens to the orchard, and to me they must be the most free-range chickens in Belgium: they can scratch around the whole day in the orchard where we also have three donkeys roaming around. The botanical value of a high-stem fruit tree orchard is important but the animal life around it is key. High-stem fruit tree orchards are a lot less vulnerable to diseases and pests because of their complete ecosystem in comparison to low-stem varieties. This means no insecticides are needed either.

Since creating Verger du Nord, I have witnessed several people in my circle of friends begin to plant heritage trees and even dive into the world of beekeeping. I really want to believe in a pollinating role I can play and to inspire people to do the same and plant native trees and plants. You do not need a big farm like I have to plant beautiful fruit trees and contribute to agricultural heritage for generations to come. I am fascinated by the history of fruit trees and love to pass on the message.

SOCIAL RESPONSIBILITY

I also try to involve other parties with Verger du Nord who can benefit from it while integrating with the social aspect of running a small-scale farm. For example, all the fencing is made and put in place by an organization that employs people with learning difficulties. Meanwhile, some of the apple juice is pressed by another company that engages people who have difficulty in finding a job.

CULTIVATING AN ORCHARD

Selecting To cultivate an orchard, everything starts with selecting the perfect heritage fruit trees. If you select well, you can have an orchard that produces fruit all year round. Some cherry trees can be harvested from mid-June, then plums are ready, pears can be picked from August, and apples from mid-August until October. The apples and pears can be preserved until April. The key is to do a lot of research and to talk to people who are also passionate about the preservation of old fruit trees.

Planting First, we study which trees should be planted where. Some trees can withstand strong winds and some need direct sunlight. We also need to have a certain mix of trees since some trees need other trees for pollination.

Nurturing Young trees have to be closely watched the first years after planting. When they start carrying fruit in the beginning, we have to remove the young apples or pears so the tree can focus all its energy on growing the roots and stem rather than producing fruit.

Pruning Pruning the trees is key to having strong and productive trees in the future. We use different pruning techniques for different fruit trees and during different times in the year. The first five years are crucial for the shape of the tree.

Picking In September it is time to pick most of the fruit. We still hand-pick and collect the fruit in small wooden crates, which are then transported to the presser. Some varieties carry more one year and almost nothing the next. For example, a French adult Bellefleur high-stem apple tree can carry up to 1000 kg per tree in one season.

Producing For the moment we outsource the pressing since the production is still too small to press myself. We store apple juice in glass bottles and we also press a batch of apples so we have unpasteurized apple juice, perfect to use for apple cider. So far, we have four wooden barrels of cider resting in the ancient stables of the farm. Towards the end of September or early October, we also transform a batch of apples and pears into apple and pear cider vinegar.

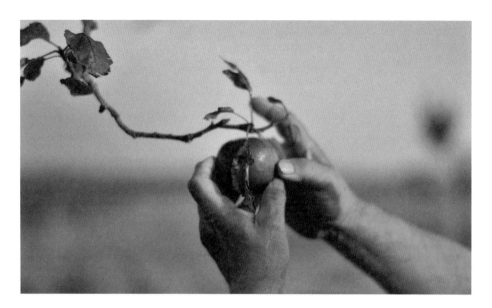

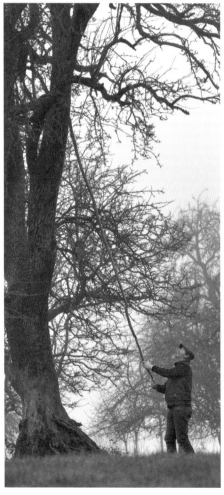

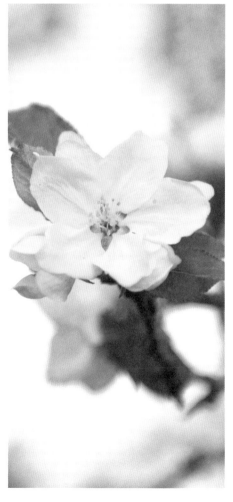

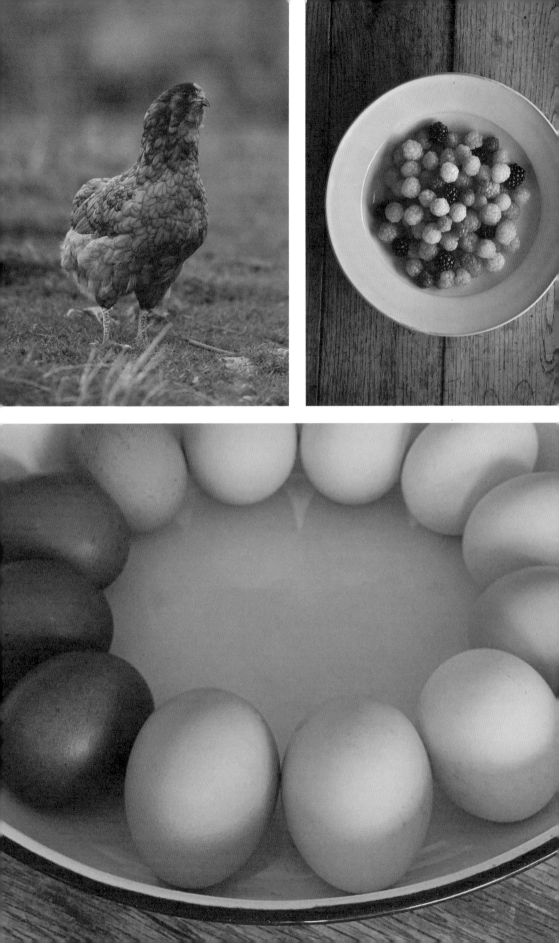

COLLABORATING WITH CHEFS

At present, I do not sell online or directly to the consumer but only to chefs who like to support us and love to work with unique products such as Verger du Nord apple juice. The first collaboration was with the 2-star Michelin restaurant The Jane in Antwerp, where chef Nick Brill served the apple juice as a shot with one of his dishes. Currently, we have a close collaboration with Graanmarkt 13 and chef Seppe Nobels. Seppe is an ambassador for 'lost' vegetables and loves to work with pure, natural, and above all local products – serving Verger du Nord juices is therefore a perfect match. I think Verger du Nord resonates with chefs because there is a story behind the brand and farm, a story of reclaiming heritage and cultivating responsibility. Then there is the fact that the juice itself is very different from any other juice. In a restaurant it can be paired with a certain dish or product, served as a non-alcoholic drink, or used in cocktails. So far, it is quite an exclusive product because of the limited amount available. I have had requests from international chefs but we have to study these requests case by case.

"My wish is that more chefs connect more with farms and collaborate together"

So far, we have attracted customers via worth of mouth and a network of celebrity chefs, thanks to my job as a photographer. To date, social media has not played a big role and Verger du Nord still has to grow in online visibility. The idea is to expand, of course. Every year the orchards become bigger, stronger, and bear more fruit. This means that we have the opportunity to grow, with the ability to supply more chefs and customers who are interested in juices made from heirloom apples. The options are quite limitless when consumers care about what they drink. Non-alcoholic high-end alternatives for a good glass of wine or champagne are more and more in demand.

My wish is that more chefs (whether 3-star Michelin chefs or small independents) connect more with farms and collaborate together. I would recommend other small-scale farmers to go and talk to chefs to see if they can help to invest in the farm or buy directly, which might make the profit model more sustainable. The only threat is, of course, the price tag of produce coming from a small-scale farm like Verger du Nord. If you do everything manually and seasonally, the cost will be higher than a more industrialized product. It all depends on whether or not the consumer, and even the restaurant owner or chef, is willing to spend the money.

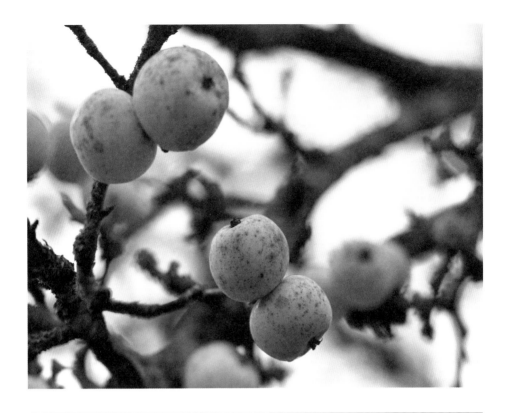

STEADY GROWTH

For the moment, however, it is not possible to earn a full salary from the farm's activities due to the many responsibilities I have. The goal is that all money generated by the orchard can sustain the running of the old farm, which needs constant love and care throughout the year. All profits we make go directly back into the orchard or into the farm, so I can't really speak of making a lot of profit with this business. The fact that I still have my full-time job as a photographer makes it possible for me to invest time and energy in the farm without making a big salary out of it.

Our production of natural apple and pear juice is still small scale, so we are not currently able to respond to high demands. It is a matter of growing until we arrive at a comfortable level where we can produce enough to make the farm sustainable again.

It is also important to keep in mind that the business grows with the expansion and the cultivation of the orchard. We cannot speed the process up since the trees decide what can be produced and sold. Some varieties only begin to bear fruit after ten years. In a way this is quite a beautiful concept, albeit not the most commercial one.

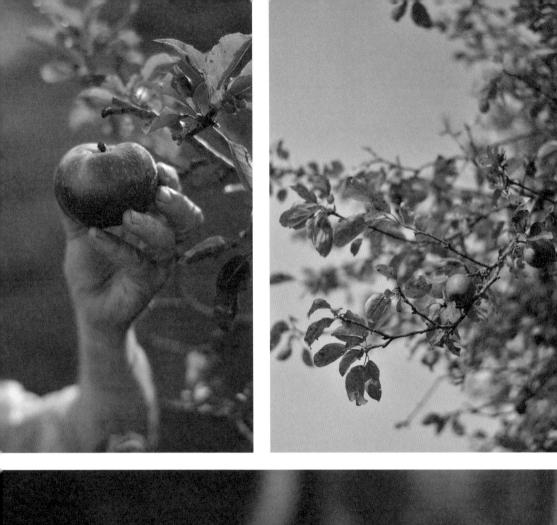
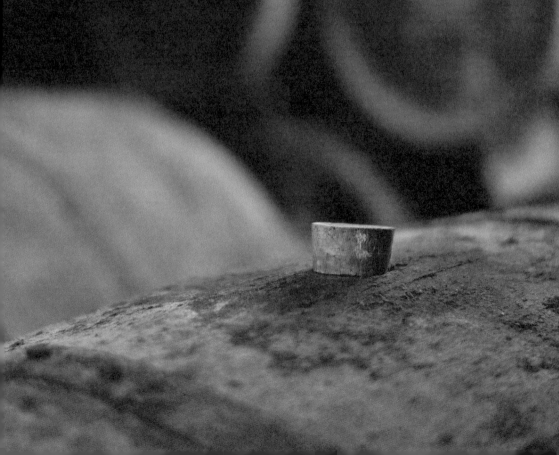

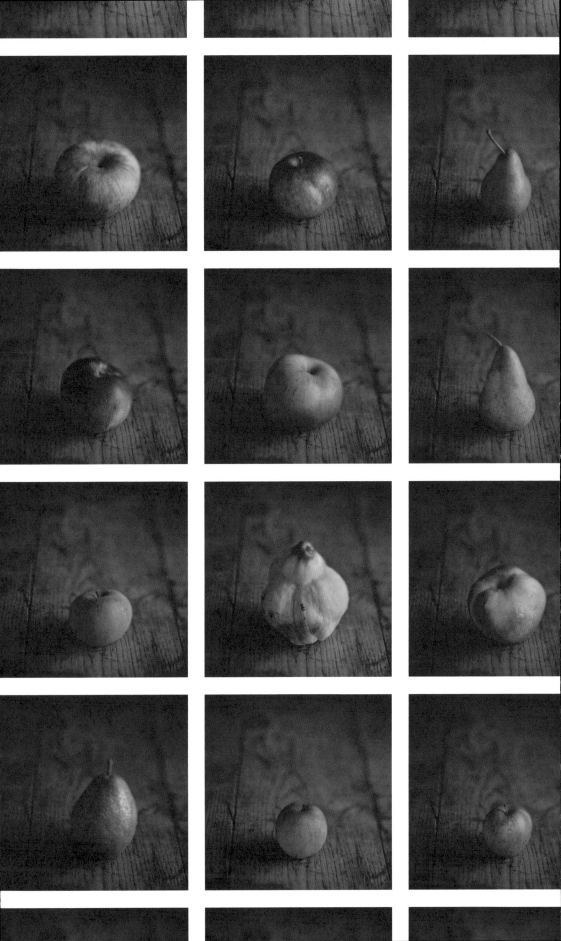

PRESERVING THE FUTURE

Of course, we can produce and sell side products on the farm. We have amazing honey and tons of walnuts coming from age-old walnut trees planted by my great-grandfather. We started making *nocino*, a sweet liquor made from unripe walnuts and originating from Italy, and we also experimented with cold-pressing walnut oil. However, this is small-scale production and more of an experiment to see if we can produce more in the future.

Together with a restaurant owner we are also planning to introduce a local breed of cow to the farm, which will be exclusively grass fed. The biggest challenge is to keep the farm operational and running as the business grows, and to find customers who believe in quality products rather than cheaper and mass-produced alternatives.

That taken into account, I find the whole production process interesting and it is mostly in September and October that I need to be on site regularly, but for the rest of the year the trees are fine without me. The fun thing about Verger du Nord is that it is multidimensional when it comes to satisfaction, from giving the farm a new purpose, to contributing to the environment by planting trees and introducing heritage varieties to Belgium, helping to create jobs, and producing healthy and natural apple juices. In the end, the whole process of finding the right trees, watching over them while they grow, and seeing them bear beautiful fruit after a few years is very rewarding.

> "If you think about the fact that humans have always gone out and gathered or hunted food, then the concept of growing your own is just magical"

It is a shame that some countries are not too careful with maintaining green zones and planting new trees. On the contrary, almost every week, more trees are cut down in favour of bio-mass energy or other reasons. It is in our hands to keep planting trees, and if we choose heirloom fruit trees we not only create better and cleaner air but also contribute to the natural heritage of a region.

I do not think Verger du Nord will ever become a very big business in terms of mass production because our philosophy is to keep it small and high quality, perfectly made for people who are not too worried about a price tag that is slightly higher than any carton of processed juice in the supermarket. The emphasis will always be on high-quality products not necessarily made for mass consumption. We should all consume less but better, and when you start planting and growing your own food, you become more conscious of the options and the difference between bad and good food. At no point in history has food been so easy to find, and in many ways, this is not such a bad thing. But if you think about the fact that humans have always gone out and gathered or hunted food, then the concept of growing your own is just magical. Once you get a taste of crafting your own food or drinks, there is no going back.

FOOD WASTE

So far in this book we have focused on the importance of provenance, supporting nature and communities, and alternative methods to industrial-scale farming. However, in addition to the early phases of the food system we should also look at the latter stages – what happens to food when we don't eat it? Statistics on food waste offer a shocking insight into how many of us view food as something cheap and inconsequential that can simply be thrown away. If we changed our perception of food and policy followed suit, it could have a massive impact on the demand for food and the cost of food production on the planet. In this section, Tristram Stuart and Toast Ale offer an innovative way of trying to tackle the food waste problem by increasing awareness of the food waste issue and proposing an alternative way of utilizing one particular waste product.

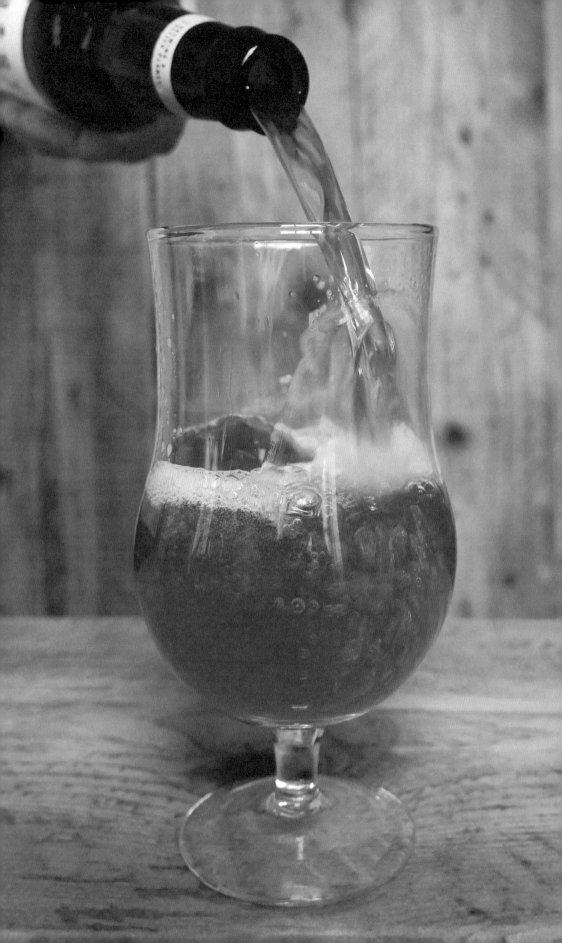

ALE

For thousands of years, ale has been a staple drink in the United Kingdom. This sweet and complex beer used to provide us with a huge percentage of our grain intake. It has similar ingredients to lager but it is fermented at a higher temperature, which is why it has a full-bodied, fruity taste and a distinctive character.

"The most ancient beer was brewed using leftover grains of bread. It is a way of preserving. Fermentation isn't principally about getting inebriated; it is about preserving the calories that would otherwise go back into something that is then stable indefinitely"

Tristram Stuart, Toast Ale

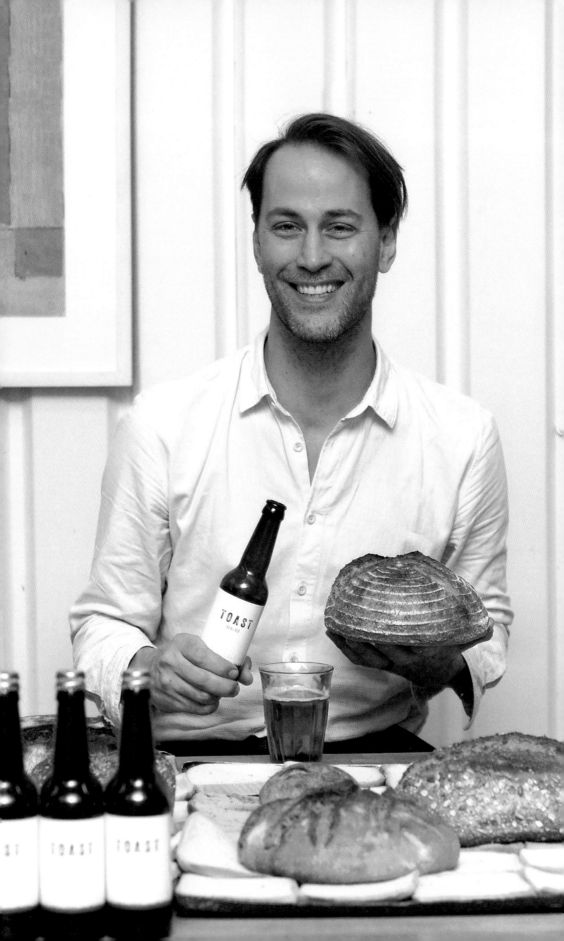

TOAST ALE

TRISTRAM STUART

London, UK | toastale.com

In 2013, I founded the environmental campaigning organization, Feedback, which is a registered UK charity. For many years in my campaigning work, I have been converting food that would otherwise be wasted into delicious drinks and meals, as a way of using food to communicate the problems of food waste and potential solutions. That is the power of food – food waste is a problem but we can turn it into delicious ways of getting the message out there. I had helped many small start-ups turning fruit and vegetables into chutneys, or jams, or juices, but it wasn't until I met the Brussels Beer Project in Belgium that I discovered that you can use bread to make beer.

Bread is one of the most wasted foods of all. I had been visiting industrial bakers and sandwich manufacturers for many years and seeing tonnes and tonnes of day-fresh, perfectly good bread being wasted every single day. Part of the system of sandwich manufacture is that the heel of every loaf that is thrown away is still fresher than the bread you can buy at the supermarket. I thought:

- Bread is being wasted all over the world.

- Craft brewing has become a global movement.

- I have spent twenty years building a food waste movement globally.

Why not unite these three phenomena together and make a business that converts the wasted bread into something that can generate revenue for the not-for-profits that are campaigning to reduce food waste, instead of being a massive burden to everyone? That is exactly what we did.

THE FOOD WASTE PROBLEM

I first became aware of just how much food was being wasted when I was a teenager at school. I had decided to keep pigs and I bought a sow and started breeding from her. I didn't want to buy livestock feed because of the environmental impact but also because it was frightfully expensive. I managed to collect uneaten school dinners, unsold food from the local greengrocer and baker, cauliflower leaves from the local green market, and wonky potatoes from the local potato farmer. It was a massive bonanza for my pigs and meant I was feeding them for free and turning food waste into pork, which was hugely valuable. But what I realized was that in every link in our food system, from the farms down to our kitchens, huge amounts of perfectly good food is going to waste. I tried to meet with supermarkets and they didn't even want to talk to me about the waste, so I went round the back and found bins jam-packed with edible food. I was shocked.

"Cutting down on waste is a really easy way to reduce our impact on the environment and increase total global food availability for people who really need it"

Food production is the single biggest impact that humans have on nature. It is the single greatest source of greenhouse gas emissions – the single biggest cause of the extinction of species – and it causes soil erosion and interrupts hydrological cycles. A third of all of that impact is needless because it goes into producing food that no one actually eats; a third of all of the world's food supply is wasted.[15] Cutting down on waste is a really easy way to reduce our impact on the environment and increase total global food availability for people who really need it. The fact that we waste food on this scale is, I think, the biggest piece of evidence that we need to deny the current dominant drive within the food system – that what we require in the world right now is to produce more and more food because there are going to be nine billion people on the planet by 2050. In fact, this plan will result in environmental destruction. What we need to do is stop wasting food and to use the food resources we have much more efficiently and fairly, and that way we can make food affordable for everyone without destroying the biosphere.

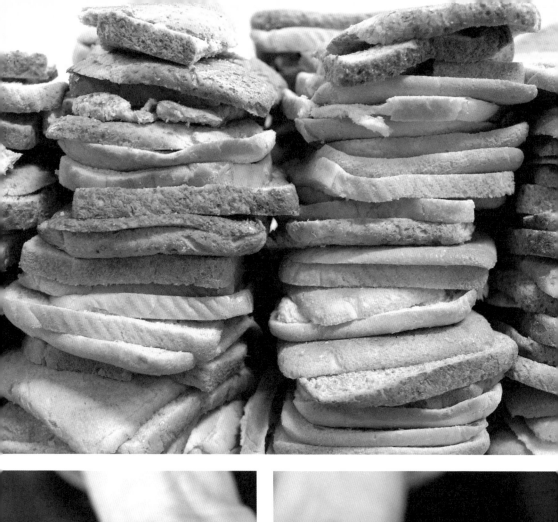

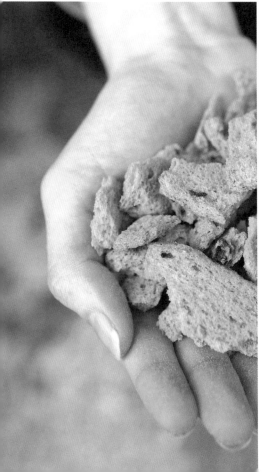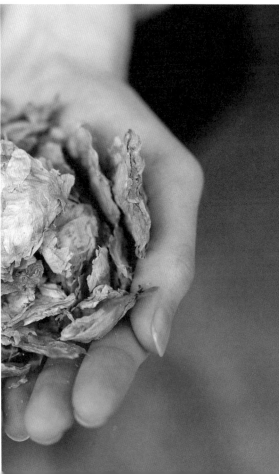

WHY DO WE WASTE SO MUCH FOOD?

One of the reasons we produce so much more food than we actually need is that it serves the economic interests of the big corporations who run the food system and run it principally as a way of making profit. I am not against profit per se, but at the moment food corporations are generating profit at the expense of both human health and the health of the environment. They do this in a number of ways. Firstly, and most obviously, the more food we as consumers buy the better as far as they are concerned – irrespective of whether we need it, whether it is good for us, or whether we are going to throw it in the bin. That is why billions of dollars are invested into marketing products like fizzy drinks that have more sugar in than is healthy to consume in a day and are laced with caffeine, a semi-addictive drug. They are out there marketing it to us, to our children, and the more of it that we buy the better: the more profit that they make.

Taking that to the supermarket system, obviously it doesn't matter as far as the supermarket is concerned that we buy more food than we actually need week after week and dump it in the bin; the money is still going to them. This goes back to the heart of our evolutionary history. Humans evolved over the last two million years in an environment of scarcity, where abundance is a rare occurrence. It made sense in those moments of cornucopia and abundance to take as much as we could, to fill our bellies, our baskets, and to go off with hoards of food. The supermarkets are tapping into that hard wired human response to abundance precisely by demonstrating a huge cornucopia on every shelf, in a high-piled visual display. That visual display prompts the human instinct to take. Our automatic response that made sense in our evolutionary history is to take more than we need. Now that we are confronted with it day after day, the result is huge and colossal food waste as well as the problem of overconsumption.

> "One of the biggest opportunities globally to help reduce environmental damage, as well as improve public health, is to rewire that food subsidy system and use public money to incentivize farmers to produce healthy food in ways that replenish and regenerate the land"

In addition to that, we have a farmer subsidy system in Europe and the USA that historically was designed to stimulate overproduction, originally for a very good reason – that of national security in order not to run out of food. That program was, by the parameter of food-surplus production, incredibly successful, and rode and subsidized the wave of advances in agricultural productivity in the second half of the twentieth century. The problem is that it has come at the expense of the environment. What we have now, particularly in the USA and to a large extent in Europe, is a system that subsidizes exactly the kinds of food that we should be eating less of: commodity crops that feed livestock to stimulate and produce more meat and dairy products. In the US, the subsidy of maize results in an industry that turns that maize not just into animal feed but also into ethanol for cars and the high-fructose corn syrup that ends up in all the sugar-filled sodas that people can become overweight on. We are using public money to pay for a farm system and to incentivize farmers to produce food in a way that harms the land and produces a food industry that harms human health.

I think one of the biggest opportunities globally to help reduce environmental damage, as well as improve public health, is to rewire that food subsidy system and use public money to incentivize farmers to produce healthy food in ways that replenish and regenerate the land, that get carbon out of the atmosphere and into the soils, that produce habitat, that help to get water back into the water table instead of causing floods and run-off. I believe that the billions of dollars and euros that are currently being misspent are among the most quick and easy opportunities we have if we can redirect that towards sustainable healthy farming.

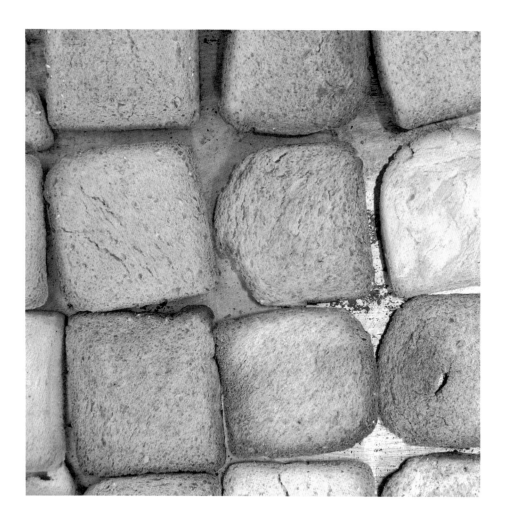

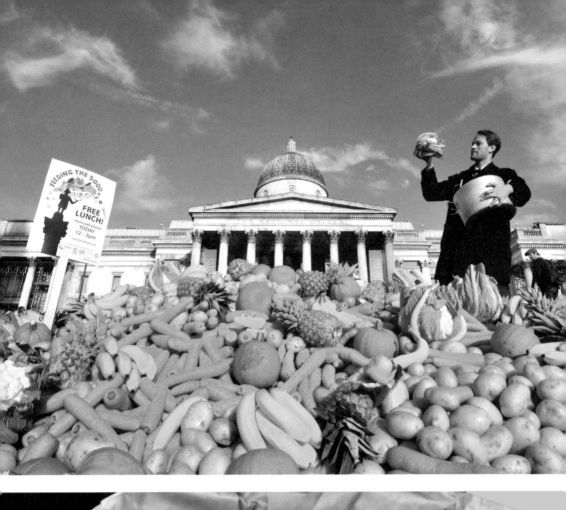

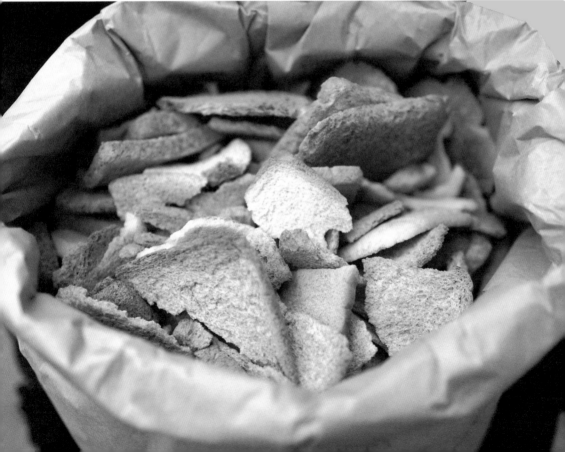

FEEDBACK

Feedback is a registered UK charity, best known for having kick-started and capitalized a vibrant global movement against food waste. I published a book on food waste in 2009 and then thought the best way of getting this message out to the wider public would be to organize an enormous feast, all made from food that would otherwise be wasted. I came up with *Feeding the 5,000* and we fed more than that many people in Trafalgar Square in December 2009. We had delicious curries and smoothies and free groceries made from wonky fruit from farmers and packers, all of which would have gone to waste. I invited all the organizations that had something to do with food waste – Consumer Awareness, charities that feed hungry people with perfectly good food surplus from the industry – and really tried to push their agenda and build a kind of movement out of the disparate parts.

The impact was immediate and enormous – we changed the policy of supermarkets. The government, who had previously done nothing about food redistribution, took on the issue. The UK Secretary of State for Environment, Food, and Rural Affairs wrote to all the CEOs of supermarkets saying they wanted them to donate food rather than destroy it. Public awareness went through the roof. It went from being a low priority to a big national priority. Everyone said you can't stop there, let's carry on. Sure enough, we started being invited by countries all over the world to replicate the launch of a vibrant national movement involving the general public and NGOs.

It began taking form around the world and we started launching lots of other campaigns. In addition to food waste, there is now campaigning on the overconsumption of meat and dairy products, which causes environmental damage, and the overconsumption of sugar, which causes environmental damage and damage to human health. Feedback is an environmental campaign group working to regenerate nature by transforming our food system. It tries to do this in an unapologetic, fact-based way, while bringing those facts to life with vibrant engagement through the use of food.

What we did with events like *Feeding the 5,000* is put a smile on people's faces while bringing them what ultimately is quite a bleak message: we are damaging our planet every day because of the way we eat and that it has been said we are in the middle of a mass species extinction such that the planet has never seen. It is really awful what is going on out there – and yet we can bring that message in a way that is inspiring and empowering and that makes people think we can turn this around, and we can do it in a way that is going to make us happy. We are going to throw a better party than whatever party we were at before. That is the motto of Toast Ale – if you want to change the world, you have to throw a better party than those destroying it. You don't clear a dance floor by walking on to the dance floor and shouting at everyone 'you're making too much noise, stop!' No, you shut down a party by saying 'hey, there's a much bigger and better party going on down the road – come and join us.'

CREATING TOAST ALE

Toast Ale is a social enterprise and certified B-Corporation. Our core product is beneficial to the environment because it uses a third less grain than conventional beer to produce. If you had a car that used a third less fuel but in all other respects was as good to drive, you would almost say it was immoral to drive any other car. The same goes for Toast Ale.

I set up Toast Ale, having worked for many years for the charity that I founded, as a way of turning this colossal problem of bread waste in the UK into a potential revenue source.[16] Raising money for charity is a constant challenge. Philanthropy has a role but I thought it would be much nicer if we could earn our own money. I therefore set up the company in such a way that one hundred per cent of the distributable profit (profit that normally ends up as dividends) goes to Feedback. In addition to that, wherever we are brewing under licence in overseas countries – Brazil, Iceland, Sweden, South Africa, and Ireland – we partner with a local not-for-profit with an aligned mission and we give them a percentage of pre-profit revenue, in addition to the distributable profit we give Feedback.

WHAT IS A B-CORPORATION?

A B-Corporation (or B-Corp) is a business that is certified as having top standards of social and environmental performance. Public transparency and the balance of profit and purpose are also taken into account as criteria in the verification process, with the idea being that the business is used as a force for good.

When the Toast Ale team proposed that we become a B-Corp, I was quite dismissive. I thought we didn't need to be a B-Corp as we were already so ethical we didn't need another organization to tell us that. Actually, the rigour of going through the B-Corp requirements was such a good discipline and put issues on our radar that would not have been put into action quite so quickly, for example in terms of company stock, welfare, and fairness in the workplace – all of these things that one might already have the will and desire that the company do, but unless all the measures are put in place they could easily not happen. It was a fantastic way of helping us align our company with what we always wanted it to be. There is a brilliant community of like-minded companies and great resources to help you do that.

BLOOMIN' LOVELY

The early days were the most fun. I had worked with Jamie Oliver on a television programme where he had covered the issue of food waste – *Friday Night Feast*. In the third series there was going to be a food-waste theme in each episode. I mentioned that we were going to start brewing beer using waste bread. The programme team were excited.

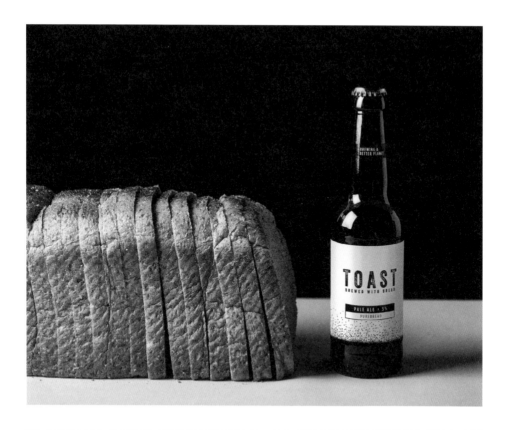

The Toast Ale team and I met with the Brussels Beer Project people. However, we had also just returned from a trip to Peru and only had thirteen days until Jamie Oliver was available to come to what was going to be our first brew – and at this point didn't have a brewery or a specified source for the bread. My assistant called round all the breweries in Hackney, which is where the charity office is headquartered. Pretty much all of them said they were interested, but one was really keen, loved the social mission, was super enthusiastic about it, and makes really good beer, so we decided to work with them. We then called round the bakery companies. Bread was donated by approximately ten bakeries from all over London, and sliced and dried at E5 Bakehouse. I then invited a representative over from the Brussels Beer Project to develop a beer that would be suitable for British tastes.

Thirteen days later, we were in the brewery with loads of surplus bread. My assistant was walking down the street, two-year-old child in one hand and a baby on her chest, also carrying a sack of bread. The team and I put the brew on. We brewed and bottled an ale that had never been drunk by anyone, and which Jamie Oliver then sampled on *Friday Night Feast*. We were so nervous! He said it was 'bloomin' lovely'. There were also some very poker-faced beer sommeliers and beer stockists – it was when they tasted it that we thought the business was going to work. One of them held a glass of it up and said: 'This is a really classic English ale, with a couple of unusual notes, really drinkable – never mind the story – it's just a damn good beer!'

INVESTMENT AND GROWTH

When the time came for us to take on investment, convincing people to invest in the company was tricky, when conventional wisdom says you evaluate a company based on its future dividend yield; people saw it as having no value. How will this be an investment rather than a piece of philanthropy? I argued that the company would grow in value and they would be able to sell their shares with a capital gain to them further down the line. I managed to convince a group of great investors that that was the case. I made their lives even more difficult by saying that if you do make a gain through your shares, you have to sign an 'equity for good pledge', which says any gain that they made must be reinvested or donated into an organization whose core business is to save the planet. Everyone did that! We tried to make it clear that all the money going into Toast Ale was designed to perpetuate good in the economy.

At the time of writing, we have grown in the last twelve months by one hundred per cent; we just brewed our millionth slice of bread. That means that if you stacked all the bread slices we have saved on top of each other, it would be one and a half times the height of Mount Everest. We are aiming for the moon – that's the financial model.

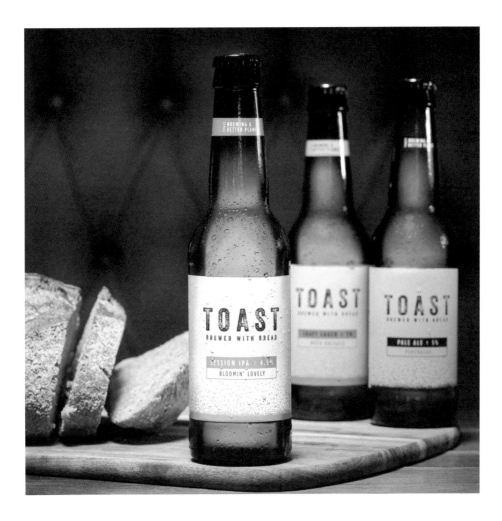

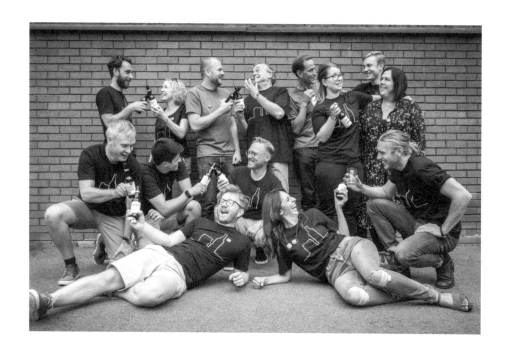

"If you want to change the world, you have to throw a better party than those destroying it"

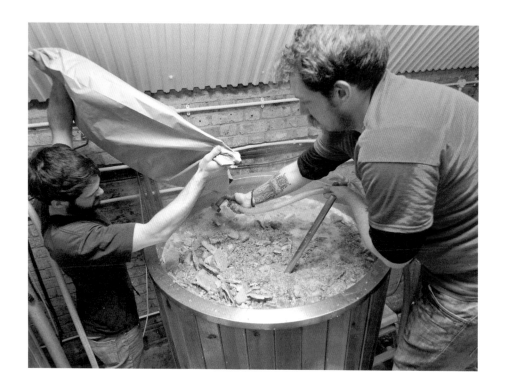

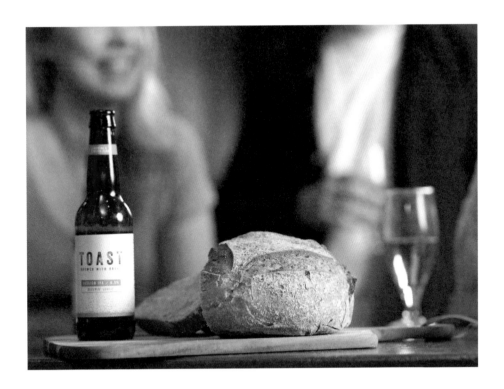

RESPONSIBLE ALCOHOL CONSUMPTION

We are bringing brewing back to its origins. The most ancient beer was brewed using leftover grains of bread. It is a way of preserving. Fermentation isn't principally about getting inebriated; it is about preserving the calories that would otherwise go back into something that is then stable indefinitely. Wine and beer are things that can be bottled up and put on the shelf for a long time because grapes, apples, and grain will not last, so we give fermentation its due in that respect.

In terms of alcohol consumption and the very real risks and dangers of it, this is something I am personally very mindful of and put good policies in place. We try to communicate the messages in a typically fun way too. Every bottle says: *Bread shouldn't be wasted and neither should you. Please drink responsibly.* I will be perfectly straightforward and say the environmental credentials of Toast Ale work if what we do is replace existing brewing with the way we brew. In other words, what we do is we go to existing brewers, using existing brewing capacity (we haven't set up our own brewery), and using bread that would otherwise be wasted to make that beer. Essentially, we see our role as a company to convert existing beer production methods to our method, because if you are going to drink beer, drink our beer as it will have less impact on the environment. As a rule, I think it's safe to say that, ultimately, we should drink less and drink better. That's really what Toast Ale is about – the solution to the world's problems is not for people to drink loads more beer. Not at all. Toast Ale is about drinking in a responsible way.

THE POTENTIAL OF INNOVATION

By supplementing barley with bread, Toast Ale has freed up the land and water otherwise used to grow thirty tonnes of barley. Growing that barley would have required seven football pitches of land and 228,768 pints of water. The land can instead be used to grow food or return to nature. By using less barley and preventing bread from going to landfill, we have also avoided emissions of 32.1 tonnes of carbon dioxide equivalent. That is the equivalent to flying around the world 9.2 times.

Toast Ale Impact Report, 2016–2018

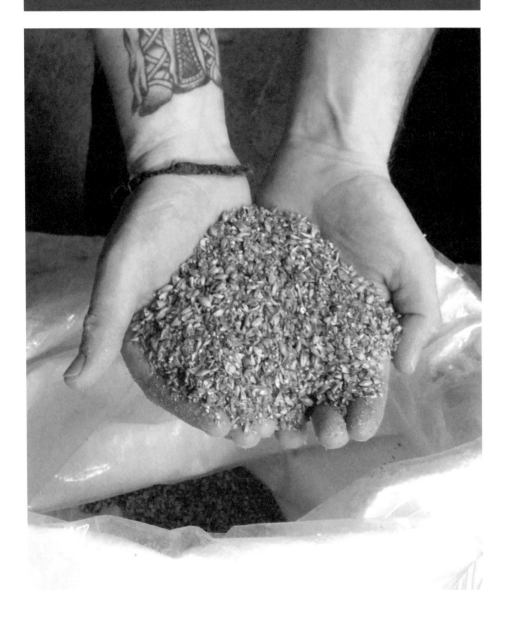

THE FUTURE

My vision for the future is that somehow the human species realizes that the survival of all species on this planet, as well as our own, depends on united and concerted action to bring an end to what is currently still an accelerating bulldozer heading in the wrong direction. The chances of succeeding in that effort are diminishing every day, but this shouldn't be a reason for despair; it should be a reason for all of us to take part in changing our everyday consumption and the way we spend our money, the way we interact with the businesses we give our money to, and the way we interact with our governments who are failing to take the action necessary to avert environmental catastrophe. If we can do that in a way that brings our fellow humans together in community, and with fun at the heart of what we do, then we can build a world that is going to be more beautiful and more fun than this incredibly lovely one that we are born into. My vision is that we achieve that and we squeeze every drop of enjoyment out of the resources and bounty and food and drink and fellow humans and other species that this wonderful world has given to us and enjoy every last bit of it to its full.

We are all empowered to reduce our food waste, to buy only what we need, and to eat everything we buy. We also need to reduce our meat and dairy consumption in a way that accords with our own health and that of the planet, and that is an individual action that anyone can engage in every day to their own level of willingness. There is no such thing as individual people acting in isolation. Humans are sociable animals; we live in community. Indeed, the very word 'companion' etymologically breaks into 'com', Latin for with, and 'pan' which is bread; a companion is someone you share bread with, who you share food with. It is by sharing food that we build companionship, that we build friendship, that we build community – at a local level by sharing food with our immediate families, friends, and neighbours, but also, more intangibly, at a global level. We are failing to realize the potential of food as the builder of companionship globally. When we waste a third of the world's food, that isn't just a waste of resources, it's a waste of potential friendship. Think of how many friends we could make with the 1.3 billion tonnes of food we waste every year if, instead of wasting, it we share it and built companionship with it. I would say that as individuals what we can do is build companionship with fellow people and connect to each other and, through food, connect to the natural world to produce that food and cherish it.

"We are all empowered to reduce our food waste, to buy only what we need, and to eat everything we buy"

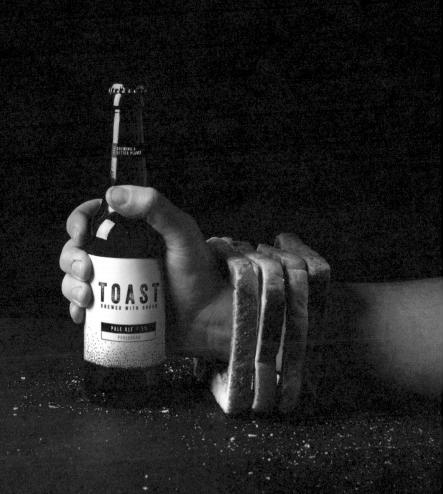

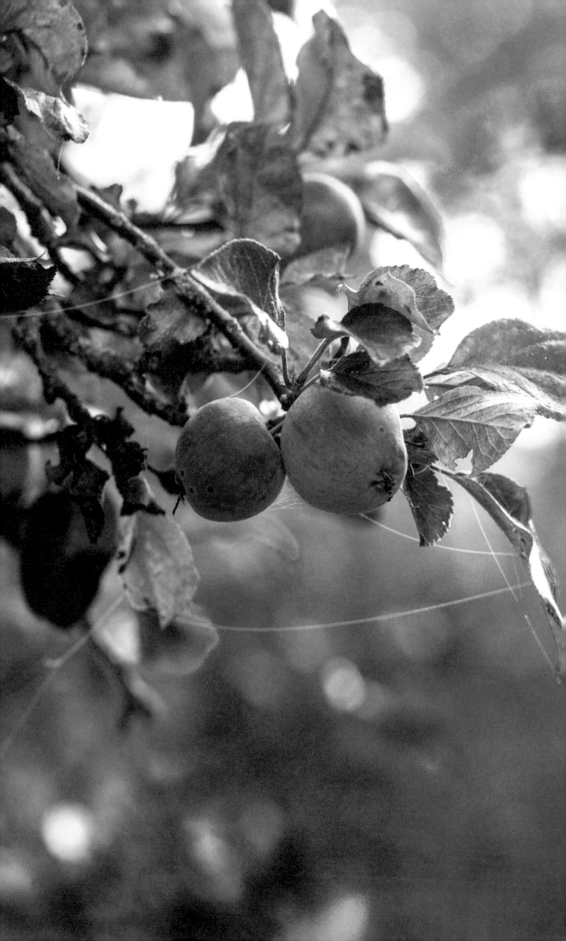

"Working with your hands, carrying out iterative processes, and doing them over and over again, edges out any sort of anxiety that you might have; it can quiet any questions of purpose or meaning in your life"

Big Island Coffee Roasters

ENDNOTES

What am I eating?

1 In this book the use of 'organic' generally refers to produce or producers who are certified organic by official certification bodies, such as the Soil Association. However, it is also used to refer to 'organic matter' in the context of things like compost, where the nutrients from naturally occurring microorganisms and processes improve soil health. The use of 'organic methods' or 'organic principles' refers to where organic techniques are followed but the producer is not necessarily certified.

2 https://www.fibl.org/en/switzerland/research/soil-sciences/bw-projekte/dok-trial.html – a thirty-five year field trial in Switzerland.

3 Slow Food Movement. https://www.slowfood.org.uk/about/about/what-we-do/

Cheese

4 H.R.J. Van Kernebeek, S.J. Oosting, M.K. Van Ittersum, P. Bikker, and I.J.M. De Boer. 'Saving Land to Feed a Growing Population: Consequences for Consumption of Crop and Livestock Products'. *The International Journal of Life Cycle Assessment* 21, no. 5 (2016), pp. 677–687.

J.O. Karlsson and E. Röös. 'Resource-efficient Use of Land and Animals – Environmental Impacts of Food Systems Based on Organic Cropping and Avoided Food-feed Competition'. *Land Use Policy* 85 (June 2019), pp. 63–72.

H.H.E.Van Zanten, M.K.Van Ittersum, and I.J.M. De Boer. 'The Role of Farm Animals in a Circular Food System'. *Global Food Security* 21 (June 2019), pp. 18–22.

5 G. Myhre, D. Shindell, F.-M. Bréon, W. Collins, J. Fuglestvedt, J. Huang, D. Koch, J.-F. Lamarque, D. Lee, B. Mendoza, T. Nakajima, A. Robock, G. Stephens, T. Takemura, and H. Zhang. 'Anthropogenic and Natural Radiative Forcing'. In *Climate Change 2013: The Physical Science Basis. Contribution of Working Group I to the Fifth Assessment Report of the Intergovernmental Panel on Climate Change*, edited by Stocker, T.F., D. Qin, G.-K. Plattner, M. Tignor, S.K. Allen, J. Boschung, A. Nauels, Y. Xia, V. Bex and P.M. Midgley. Cambridge, UK: Cambridge University Press, 2013.

6 C. Opio, P. Gerber, A. Mottet, A. Falcucci, G. Tempio, M. MacLeod, T. Vellinga, B. Henderson, and H. Steinfeld. *Greenhouse Gas Emissions from Ruminant Supply Chains – A Global Life Cycle Assessment.* Rome: Food and Agriculture Organization of the United Nations (FAO), 2013.

C. Rasmussen. 'NASA-led Study Solves a Methane Puzzle'. 2018. https://climate.nasa.gov/news/2668/nasa-led-study-solves-a-methane-puzzle/

7 In agriculture, a co-product comes from the primary production of a crop, like straw in a cereal crop.

8 A by-product is produced from the waste from the manufacture of a food product, like soybean meal from the production of soya oil, or dark grains from the production of whisky.

9 An arable rotation is a crop rotation which includes arable crops, such as wheat, oilseed rape, or potatoes, for which the ground needs to be ploughed before sowing. These nutrient-hungry crops are grown only for a year or two, after which grass, clover, and other forage crops are sown and grazed by livestock, allowing soil fertility to build up again. The use of artificial fertilizer can allow farmers to dispense with crop rotation and grow the same arable crop continuously. This leads to the loss of soil-organic carbon with the knock-on effects of soil erosion, water run-off leading to flooding, and the collapse of soil structure. The inclusion of a grass break of two or three years with grazing livestock re-builds that soil organic matter.

Kefir
10 A UK food standards scheme that covers animal welfare, food safety, traceability and environmental protection.

Honey
11 *London: Garden City?* Research project by Chloë Smith on behalf of London Wildlife Trust, Greenspace Information for Greater London, and the Greater London Authority, 2010.

Chocolate
12 Agroforestry is a practice of agroecology where trees and crops or pastureland are integrated. This technique is associated with a number of benefits including increasing biodiversity, reducing soil erosion, and offering shade to livestock, which results in the animals requiring less energy to remain cool and therefore less food.

Coffee
13 Hydroponics is a technique of raising crops without using soil, instead supplying mineral nutrients dissolved in water.

Gin
14 In distillation, the middle cut is the heart of the spirit, achieved after all impurities are distilled out and the alcohol level has been reduced to the desired percentage.

Ale
15 Food and Agriculture Organization of the United Nations (FAO). *Global Food Losses and Food Waste – Extent, Causes and Prevention.* Rome: FAO, 2011.

16 In 2012 The Waste and Resources Action Programme (WRAP) reported that 24 million whole slices of bread are thrown away every day in UK. WRAP. 'Household Food and Drink Waste in the United Kingdom'. 2012. Available from wrap.org.uk

ACKNOWLEDGEMENTS

Opening pages	pp. 3, 7, 8 © David de Vleeschauwer, www.classetouriste.com; p. 4 © Simon Morse
Foreword	All photos Rob Baker Ashton @robbakerashton
What am I eating?	pp. 16, 37 (top and bottom), 38 (all images), 41 (middle right) © Beau Cacao
	p. 19 (top) © 3dtotal.com Ltd
	p. 19 (bottom) Adobe Stock © pressmaster
	pp. 20, 24 (bottom), 35 (bottom) © Charles Dowding
	p. 21 © Big Island Coffee Roasters
	pp. 23, 24 (top), 35 (top) by Caitlin Tyler © Chuckling Goat
	pp. 27 and 34 © Cooking for Sanity
	pp. 28 (top), 29 © Simon Morse
	p. 28 (bottom) Rowland Roques-O'Neil @roquesoneilphoto
	pp. 30–31 Adobe Stock © hroephoto
	pp. 33 (top and bottom), 41 (bottom left) © David de Vleeschauwer, www.classetouriste.com
	p. 41 (top and bottom right) Ian Findlay www.findlaydesign.co.uk © Ethical Dairy
Cheese	All photos Ian Findlay www.findlaydesign.co.uk © Ethical Dairy
Kefir	All photos by Caitlin Tyler © Chuckling Goat
Honey	p. 95 © 3dtotal.com Ltd
	All other photos Rowland Roques-O'Neil @roquesoneilphoto
Apple cider vinegar	All photos © Willy's Ltd

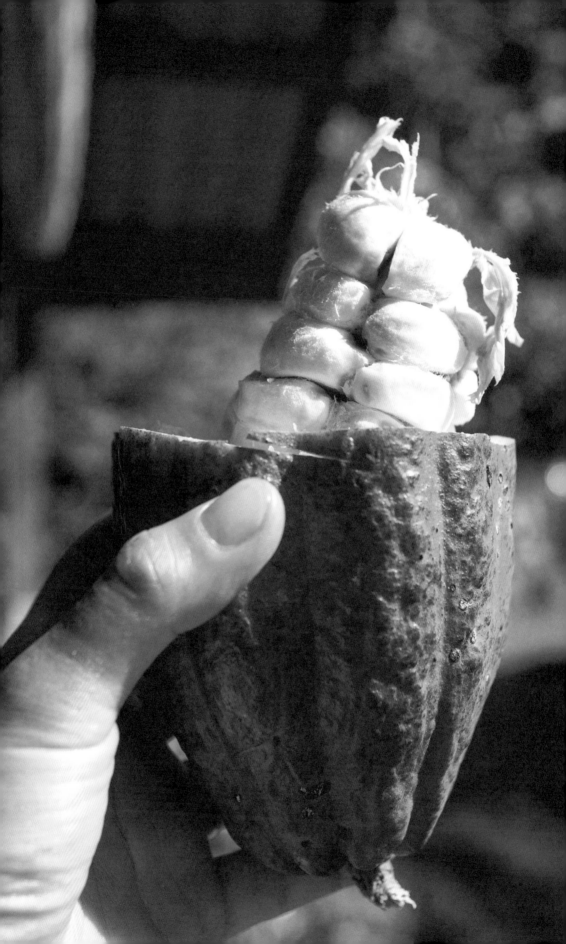

"Every pound, euro, or dollar you spend is a vote for a better ecosystem"

Beau Cacao

WORN & WORN

WOVEN & WORN

GATHER & NOURISH

FORGE & CARVE

THE SEARCH FOR WELL-BEING AND SUSTAINABILITY IN THE MODERN WORLD

"I do what I do because of the generosity of others who shared their knowledge freely and I am more than happy to do the same"

Éamonn O'Sullivan | Spoon carver | hewn.ie
Forge & Carve

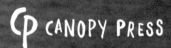

canopy-press.com | instagram.com/canopypress